The
MIND
Diet

The MIND Diet

A Scientific Approach to Enhancing Brain Function and Helping Prevent Alzheimer's and Dementia

MAGGIE MOON, MS, RDN

Foreword by Sharon Palmer, RDN
author of *The Plant-Powered Diet*

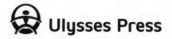 Ulysses Press

Published in the United States by:
Ulysses Press
P.O. Box 3440
Berkeley, CA 94703
www.ulyssespress.com

ISBN13: 978-1-61243-607-4
Library of Congress Control Number: 2016934497

Printed in the United States by United Graphics
10 9 8 7 6 5 4 3

Acquisitions editor: Casie Vogel
Managing editor: Claire Chun
Editor: Renee Rutledge
Proofreader: Lauren Harrison
Indexer: Sayre Van Young
Front cover design: Double R Design
Cover artwork: all from shutterstock.com chicken © Photocrea; salmon © ElenaGaak; wine © Givaga; spinach © Binh Thanh Bui; berries © Volosina; olives © Gayvoronskaya_Yana; nuts and dried fruit © Valentyn Volkov
Interior design: what!design @ whatweb.com
Interior artwork: © Serg64/shutterstock.com
Layout: Jake Flaherty

Distributed by Publishers Group West

IMPORTANT NOTE TO READERS: This book has been written and published strictly for informational and educational purposes only. It is not intended to serve as medical advice or to be any form of medical treatment. You should always consult your physician before altering or changing any aspect of your medical treatment and/or undertaking a diet regimen, including the guidelines as described in this book. Do not stop or change any prescription medications without the guidance and advice of your physician. Any use of the information in this book is made on the reader's good judgment after consulting with his or her physician and is the reader's sole responsibility. This book is not intended to diagnose or treat any medical condition and is not a substitute for a physician.

This book is independently authored and published and no sponsorship or endorsement of this book by, and no affiliation with, any trademarked brands or other products mentioned within is claimed or suggested. All trademarks that appear in ingredient lists and elsewhere in this book belong to their respective owners and are used here for informational purposes only. The authors and publishers encourage readers to patronize the quality brands mentioned and pictured in this book.

For In Moon and Teju Ziggy,
the eldest and youngest bright minds in my family.

Contents

APPENDIX 255

Foreword

Fall in love with plants, and they will love you back.

Imagine this: There are more than 40,000 edible plant species on the planet, according to scientists, and within each species there are sometimes thousands of varieties. Each plant, from the rich, savory tomato to the bitter, pungent wild green, tells a story as it evolves along with mankind, developing its own unique colors, flavors, and textures—and cache of nutrients. Researchers today know that these plants are teeming with compounds called phytochemicals, which have the power to protect the plant from its threats, such as sun damage and pests. And these plants provide protection to humans too, creating a symbiotic relationship between people and plants. We care for the plants and pluck their fruits, and then cast away the seeds to start a new cycle of life; meanwhile we are sustained and nurtured by these plants as we live a long, prosperous life.

We've known for some time that many whole plants—including leafy greens, berries, beans, nuts, whole grains, wine, and olives—are protective against many chronic diseases of our time, including cardiovascular disease and type 2 diabetes. So it comes as no surprise that the same list of foods—along with fish—appears to be good for the brain too. These foods are packed with brain-loving compounds, including carotenoids, flavonoids, and omega-3 fatty acids. By focusing on these foods, you crowd out the foods in your diet that appear to be troublesome for human health, such as red meat, saturated fats, and highly processed foods.

Why is this eating style protective for the brain? Though we need more research in this area, studies have shown that Mediterranean-style eating patterns are linked with a lower risk of neurodegenerative diseases, and now the MIND diet has been shown to protect against cognitive decline in aging. The MIND diet combines a Mediterranean diet with Dietary Approaches to Stop Hypertension diet (DASH)—two of the most widely studied and successful diet patterns on the planet. These also happen to be two of the diet patterns recommended by the brand new *Dietary Guidelines for Americans 2015-2020*.

I love what these two diet patterns have in common: a focus on whole, minimally processed plant foods. These foods are colorful, potent in flavor, packed with antioxidant and anti-inflammatory compounds, and rich in fiber, healthy fats, vitamins, and minerals, all of which may be key to their brain-protective abilities. Compare this to a typical American diet (also called the Western diet), which is high in animal foods, highly processed foods, sugar, and salt, and low in whole plant foods; thus, it is pitifully poor in all of those compounds we know to be health-protective. No wonder scientists think that the Western diet may be linked to Alzheimer's disease, and an estimated 25 percent of cases may be traced back to diet and inactivity. Alzheimer's is more prevalent in developed countries where the Western diet is more prominent—the US is among the top three countries with the highest Alzheimer's rates. Studies have even shown that people who migrate to the US have higher rates of the disease compared to those still living in their native homelands—highlighting that Alzheimer's may be more strongly related to environment and lifestyle, rather than just genetics.

What's more, the MIND diet is an eating pattern that will nourish your whole body—heart, kidney, muscles, brain, and beyond. And it's also better for the planet. As we move away from highly processed diets packed with red meat, we also reduce our carbon and water footprint. Best of all, this style of eating is delicious! Savory, fleshy beans; sautéed greens in lemon and olive oil; spiced, crunchy farro; fresh berries dusted with chopped walnuts; a glass of red wine. Does that sound hard? Indeed, I believe that one of the main reasons we find benefits surrounding the Mediterranean and DASH diet patterns is that they are delicious and easy to sustain. Unlike many fad diets, which leave you hungry and deprived, these diet patterns are focused on fulfillment and good health. With a focus on real, flavorful foods, spices, olive oil, a touch of dark chocolate, and a glass of wine, you can feel truly good about this way of eating. And what's good for the body and soul—in this case—is also good for the mind.

I'm very excited about this fabulous book, which explains the very core of the MIND diet, written by my friend and colleague Maggie Moon, MS, RDN. Maggie is a talented dietitian, so skilled and practiced at crafting the latest evidence on nutrition science into an easy-to-digest, attainable method of eating for life. She has created a veritable blueprint for a healthy way of eating, for your mind *and* whole body. Let Maggie be your personal dietitian as she guides you through these pages, offering you a glimpse of how a healthy mind operates and which foods will best fuel your brain. Follow her practical tips and try out her delicious recipes in order to put the MIND diet into practice every single day. Make a smarter move toward cognitive health with every bite.

—Sharon Palmer, RDN,
    author of *The Plant-Powered Diet* and *Plant-Powered for Life*,
    www.sharonpalmer.com

Preface

Dear Reader,

This book is about eating right to keep your brain young and healthy. The recommendations within this book are based on a substantial body of science. The MIND diet refers to the Mediterranean-dietary approaches to stop hypertension (DASH) Intervention for Neurodegenerative Delay. It is based on years of cumulative research findings on which foods and nutrients benefit and harm brain function. Not only that, it is built upon a foundation of two proven diets that have been studied for many decades and practiced, in good health, for centuries.

Because this diet is based on research, I do spend time explaining the science. While this can get a bit technical at times, this is not meant to be a textbook. More useful for you, reader, is that it's a practical guide to crafting delicious and nourishing snacks, meals, and eating plans using the latest science in diet and dementia.

As a registered dietitian nutritionist (RDN), my goal is to be the bridge between the science and the plate. There aren't a lot of resources available for putting this important eating plan into action. That's where this book comes in. I provide tools to make it easy to keep track of your daily and weekly MIND diet points, and more than 75 delicious recipes and meal ideas to bring the MIND diet to life.

I hope you enjoy it as much as I enjoyed writing it for you.

Be well,

Maggie Moon, MS, RDN

P.S.—We are still learning about nutrition and the brain. Even the MIND diet researchers, the brains (forgive the pun) behind how to eat for cognitive health, acknowledge that there's still so much to learn. In fact, they expect to add more foods to the MIND diet as the science advances and are in the midst of a new MIND diet trial as of 2016. In the meantime, you can feel good about eating the MIND diet way, as the foods in the MIND diet align with several highly respected healthy diets.

Introduction

The happy fact is that Americans are living longer, and a long life is made better by a healthy and active mind. Cognitive decline is a growing public health concern, one where diet could play a role, just as it does in heart disease, diabetes, and obesity. There are trustworthy, research-backed diets for heart health, diabetes, and weight management, and now, the MIND diet is here for brain health. The research suggests that what you put on your plate can help or hinder cognitive abilities such as memory, language, attention, and more. This book focuses on proven ways of eating to keep the mind healthy, cognitively "younger," and less at risk of Alzheimer's disease.

The MIND diet covers 15 food groups, including five types of foods to avoid, but twice as many to enjoy. The best foods for your brain include green, leafy vegetables, nuts, beans, berries, poultry, fish, whole grains, olive oil, and wine. Avoid red meat, butter and stick margarine, whole-fat cheese, pastries and sweets, and fried fast food.

The MIND Diet will show you how easy and delicious it can be to keep your mind sharp and feel up to seven and a half years younger in cognitive age. To set the stage, Part One of this book explains the basics of the brain and mental fitness, as well as the science behind the MIND diet, in an approachable and understandable way. It summarizes the research backing the recommendations to seek or avoid certain foods and nutrients for brain health.

Next, Part Two of the book will guide you through how to create your own MIND diet plan, including what to eat, how much, and how often. Helpful worksheets for meal planning, keeping track of your progress, and overall lifestyle recommendations for brain health will be included.

Part Three brings the MIND diet to life through 75 recipes and meal ideas designed by the nation's leading nutrition experts, complete with key nutritional information. All recipes comply with the MIND diet parameters, and there are delicious and nutritious options for breakfast, mains, salads, soups, sides, snacks, spreads, beverages, and desserts.

Part Four of the book features profiles on the brain-healthy foods that form the foundation of the MIND diet, from seasonality and culinary uses to fascinating historical background. I'll provide guidance and strategies for choosing the healthiest options when confronted with foods from the brain-harming food groups. I'll also provide tip sheets to deliver practical information at a glance. There are tip sheets on kitchen shortcuts, untraditional ways to use MIND diet foods, top plant protein foods, sustainable seafood options, and simple snack pairings, as well as a quick reference to what foods are part of the MIND diet.

This book comes at a time when memory loss and cognitive decline are common and are among the greatest fears for aging adults. According to the CDC, Americans are twice as afraid of losing cognitive skills as they are about losing physical abilities, especially memory. Age-related cognitive decline can result in a loss of independence and emotional distress. That's why this book is about hope, prevention, and taking positive action today to slow cognitive decline and minimize risk of Alzheimer's disease down the road. While the science of diet for preventing Alzheimer's disease is relatively young, it is possible and probable that making long-term changes to how you eat can have a protective effect.

The even better news is that the MIND diet is the simplest way to get there because it is less demanding than the Mediterranean or Dietary Approaches to Stop Hypertension (DASH) diets that it is based on, and effective even when moderately followed.

PART ONE
The Science of the MIND Diet

CHAPTER 1
The Brain

Super-Basic Brain Overview

What follows is a very basic orientation to the brain and general cognitive functions that will be relevant in this book. It is by no means comprehensive or even very detailed. Simple information about various sections of the brain will be explained in approachable language. For example, rather than discuss the anterior and posterior brain, words like "front" and "back" will be used.

After establishing a basic framework for how the brain works, this chapter will explore how the brain changes with cognitive decline, dementia, and Alzheimer's disease.

Brain Basics

The brain has three main parts. The largest part of the brain is called the cerebrum, and it handles higher functions like reasoning, learning, emotions, speech, fine motor control, correctly interpreting touch, vision, and hearing, and of course, memory. When this book discusses the brain, it refers to the cerebrum. (For your information, the other two parts are smaller and sit under the brain. They're called the cerebellum and brain stem, and they maintain functions such as breathing, digestion, body temperature, and balance.)

The brain has two sides—left and right—called hemispheres. Each hemisphere has four sections, one in front, one in back, and two in the middle stacked on top of each other. These sections are called lobes, and there are eight total.

Each lobe is affiliated with a certain set of functions. Lobes are not independent, though. It's important to recognize that just like no man is an island, no lobe can act alone. Brain-imaging studies have shown how multiple parts of the brain are active at the same time during any given task.

The front lobe, aptly called the frontal lobe (just wait, they aren't all named with as much common sense), is the most advanced area of the brain. It receives information gathered through the senses (sight, touch, taste, hearing, smell) and spatial awareness (e.g., balance and movement), and is in charge of planning, short-term memory (working memory), understanding abstract ideas, inhibiting behaviors that may be emotionally or socially inappropriate, voluntary movement, and expressive language. These complex planning behaviors are associated with activity in the front part of the frontal lobe, called the prefrontal cortex, which lies just behind the forehead.

The lower middle lobe, called the temporal lobe, plays a major role in hearing, understanding language, memory, and learning and retaining information. There are upper, middle, and lower regions that are technically called superior, medial, and inferior. The medial temporal lobe (MTL) includes the hippocampus, which is involved with forming long-term memories and spatial navigation abilities. When it's damaged, the result is memory loss and disorientation.

The upper middle lobe is called the parietal lobe and is the key player in making sense of what the body touches. It's also involved in spatial thinking, such as rotating objects in your mind, being able to store ideas of movement, and controlling your intention to move. This part of the brain comes in handy in dance classes. Also, like the frontal lobe, it's involved in short-term memory.

The last and fourth section is at the back of the brain. This back lobe is called the occipital lobe. This area of the brain is farthest from the eyes, and yet, is the primary center for making sense of what you see. It is extremely important in vision.

Just below the back lobe is an area called the cerebellum, which is important to know because it has more neurons than any other part of the brain. It has many connections to the frontal lobe and most other areas of the brain. It's involved in learning and coordinating movement.

The Hungry Brain

The brain is the body's hungriest organ, using up more energy than any other organ—up to 20 percent of daily calories. The brain's preferred energy source is glucose, which it gets when the food we eat is broken down and some of the glucose is transported to the brain cells (neurons) through blood. It has a high metabolism and uses up nutrients quickly.

Not only is the brain hungry for energy, it's also hungry for antioxidants. The brain is particularly sensitive to oxidative stress, a result of having more free radicals, or unstable molecules that damage cells, than antioxidants to neutralize them. Oxidative stress causes damage to the brain tissue. In fact, a theory in the field of brain disorders is that the brain needs to be saved from oxidation and inflammation via antioxidants (e.g., vitamins E, C, and A, flavonoids, or plant compounds, and enzymes) and the minerals it needs to function at its best (e.g., manganese, copper, selenium, and zinc).

There are two kinds of antioxidants the body uses: enzymes made by the body and nutrients from food. The antioxidant enzymes the body creates can prevent toxic substances from being created in the first place, and antioxidant nutrients from food can neutralize the damaging consequences of oxidation, such as free radicals. The brain doesn't have as many antioxidant enzymes at its disposal as other parts of the body, which means antioxidant nutrients have a bigger role to play. This is one reason good nutrition and healthy eating is so important to maintaining a healthy brain.

The Fat Brain

Similar to the rest of the body, most of the brain is water (about 75 percent). However, take away the water and you're left with brain matter, 60 percent of which is fat (also known as lipids). Fats are an essential structural component of neurons. It's no surprise, then, that the brain needs healthy fats to function properly, from facilitating better blood flow to improving memory and mood. Neurons communicate through a signaling system that gets updated when a new supply of fatty acids is available.

The body produces all the saturated fat it needs, but some fats need to come from the diet. Namely, essential polyunsaturated omega-3 and omega-6 fats. The American diet typically supplies enough omega-6 fats, but not enough omega-3s, which come from fish, nuts, and seeds.

The most metabolically active fat in the brain is a poly-unsaturated type of fat called omega-3 docosahexaenoic acid (DHA), which is found in fatty fish like salmon. The body can also convert omega-3 alpha-linolenic acid (ALA), which comes from plant foods like flaxseed and walnuts, into DHA. That means the body doesn't technically require outside sources of DHA, but it's helpful since it only converts about half a percent of ALA to DHA.

As different fats are digested and absorbed, cholesterol is transported around the body in various forms, such as LDL cholesterol (sometimes called "bad" cholesterol) and HDL cholesterol (sometimes called "good" cholesterol). Cholesterol is an essential part of healthy cell membranes, and plays a role in hormone and vitamin D production. The role of cholesterol in Alzheimer's disease isn't fully clear, but studies have found that higher levels of LDL cholesterol was linked to more plaque in the brain associated with Alzheimer's disease (amyloid plaques).

What Is Cognition?

To understand what cognitive decline is, it's important to first identify just what cognition is. Simply put, it's thinking. But it's far from simple. Cognition affects how a person understands the world and acts within it, and it includes all the mental skills needed to carry out simple and complex tasks alike, from locking the front door to analyzing a scientific report. To elaborate, cognition is a word that describes the process of receiving sensory inputs (e.g., what we see, read, touch, taste, feel, smell, or hear), and transforming those inputs into their most important components (reduction), filling in gaps (elaboration), remembering (storing and recovering memories), and using the inputs to interact with the world around us, understand language, solve problems, and more.

According to the National Institute on Aging, a division of the National Institutes of Health in the U.S. Department of Health and Human Services:

> Cognition is the ability to think, learn, and remember. It is the basis for how we reason, judge, concentrate, plan, and organize. Good cognitive health, like physical health, is very important as we get older, so that we can stay independent and keep active. Some declines in cognition and memory with age are normal, but sometimes they can signal problems.

Cognitive abilities, or brain functions, include perception, attention, memory, motor skills, language, visuospatial processing, and executive functioning, as explained below:

- Perception is how our senses recognize and take in information. It's what happens when we receive sensory inputs.

- Attention is the ability to continue to concentrate on something while filtering out competing thoughts or sensory stimulation in the environment. It includes reduction skills.

- Memory can be short term or long term. Short-term memory can be as short as 20 seconds and might be used when reading a step in a recipe before doing it, while long-term memory is just that and stores memories for years and years.

- Motor skills, not often thought of as a cognitive ability, definitely use brain power, and the loss of these skills can be part of the challenges of cognitive decline. These are the skills used to move our muscles (e.g., tap dance, patting your head while rubbing your stomach at the same time, walking) and manipulate objects (e.g., leveraging a tennis racket, using a pencil) at will.

- Language skills are what allow our brains to understand (translate sounds into words) and use language (generate verbal responses).

- Visuospatial skills include the ability to see objects and understand the spatial relationship between them. For example, being able to tell how far apart two pencils are when placed near each other, and whether they are lying at the same or different angles. These skills are also used when mentally rotating a shape.

- Executive functioning can also be thought of as reasoning skills, and includes the ability to plan and do things. These abilities include using flexible thinking modes, empathetically imagining what someone else likes or dislikes, anticipating an outcome based on past experience, identifying a problem and finding solutions, making choices, using short-term memory to receive information just long enough to use it (working memory), being self-aware of emotions enough to manage them, breaking down complex ideas or actions into small steps and putting them in the right order of what needs to get done first (chef's use this in their mise en place, the process of reviewing a recipe and executing it in the right order), and focusing in a manner that can eliminate inner and outer distractions.

What Is Cognitive Decline?

Why does cognitive ability decline with age? Age-related cognitive decline is described as "normal," while mild cognitive impairment (MCI) or the more serious neurodegenerative conditions of dementia or Alzheimer's disease are differentiated from normal changes.

Normal changes could include a gradual decline in conceptual reasoning (this explains why older adults tend to think more concretely than younger adults), memory (e.g., forgetting facts and dates, having a hard time recalling recently learned information), and processing speed (e.g., slower response to a green light).

According to a recent review of neuroscience research that appeared in a 2013 issue of *Clinics in Geriatric Medicine*, the normal aging brain may show signs of cognitive wear and tear due to a loss of gray matter volume and changes to white matter. Gray matter fills 40 percent of the brain and white matter fills the remaining 60 percent. Gray matter is where all the processing goes on; white matter allows different gray areas to communicate with one another and with other parts of the body. If gray matter is like a factory, then white matter is the truck that transports goods from one factory to another, or from one factory to a store. It seems that when it comes to age-related cognitive decline, the issue is not black and white, it's gray and white.

As a part of normal aging, the amount of gray matter starts to go down after age 20, especially in the prefrontal cortex, but also in the hippocampus. Scientists believe this decrease might be due to dying neurons. A protein called beta-amyloid, which has been found in all people with Alzheimer's dementia, can kill neurons. Beta-amyloid is also found in 20 to 30 percent of normal adults, which may, but doesn't necessarily, predict that they'll ever develop Alzheimer's disease. Another explanation is that neurons grow smaller and the number of connections between them also decreases. These decreases are very well documented in older adults. With aging, neurons become simpler, shorter, and less connected to other neurons.

White matter shrinks much more than gray matter as we get older. Similar areas of the brain have shown 16 to 20 percent losses of white matter but only 6 percent of gray matter loss. The results of these normal changes to the brain over time are small and shouldn't get in the way of daily activities.

MCI is more serious than age-related cognitive decline. It is a condition that affects memory and thinking (e.g., planning, organizing, judgment) enough that it's noticeable, but not to the point that it interferes with daily life. Some causes of cognitive impairment, such as medication side effects, vitamin B12 deficiency, and depression, are treatable. MCI is a risk factor for Alzheimer's disease, but having mild cognitive impairment doesn't always lead to Alzheimer's disease.

What Is Dementia?

Dementia literally means "without mind" (de = without; mentia = mind). Dementia is a set of symptoms but not a disease of its own. It's a term used to describe symptoms that can be caused by brain disorders such as Alzheimer's disease or a stroke. Symptoms of dementia include problems with memory, thinking, language, or social skills, and uncharacteristic behavior changes. Aging doesn't cause dementia, though dementia is more common in older adults.

The occasional forgetfulness, having trouble recalling a word, or any of these symptoms could be a normal part of aging without being related to dementia. The difference is when the symptoms start to get in the way of everyday life, or activities of daily living (ADL); for example, when symptoms become disruptive to working, getting dressed, or making meals.

Examples of ADL:

Bathing—washing yourself, including getting in and out of the tub or shower.

Dressing—putting on and taking off clothes, shoes, braces, artificial limbs.

Going to the toilet—getting to and from, on and off, and using the toilet.

Getting around the house—sometimes called transferring. This refers to getting in and out of bed, chairs, or a wheelchair.

Continence—being able to control bowel and bladder functions.

Eating—eating and drinking enough to meet nutritional needs.

Other examples—using the telephone, shopping, preparing food, housekeeping, doing laundry, operating a mode of transportation, having responsibility for own medication, and having the ability to handle finances.

By mid-century, approximately a quarter of the US population will be 65 years and older, and more than one in three of this older population will likely develop dementia. The rate of dementia rises drastically with advancing years; the rate is 3 percent among 65 to 74 year olds, 19 percent among 75 to 84 year olds, and 47 percent among those 85 years old and up.

There are over 50 different conditions associated with dementia, but the most common cause of dementia is Alzheimer's disease, which accounts for 60 to 80 percent of all cases of dementia. Lewy body disease (abnormal protein clumps in brain cells), hardening arteries (arteriosclerosis) in the brain, and stroke are also common causes of dementia. Other diseases that can cause the symptoms of dementia are Parkinson's disease, Huntington's disease, HIV infection, head injury, severe depression, and Creutzfeldt-Jakob disease.

There are also nondisease causes of dementia symptoms. The National Institutes of Health indicates that dementia-like symptoms could be the result of medications, metabolic problems, nutritional deficiencies, infections, poisoning, brain tumors, lack of oxygen to the brain, and heart and lung problems.

Most dementias are irreversible. However, there are exceptions to this rule. Some forms of dementia can be stopped or even reversed if caught soon enough. These include dementia-like symptoms caused by vitamin deficiencies, brain tumors, chronic alcoholism, and some medications.

What Is Alzheimer's Disease?

Alzheimer's disease is the most common cause of dementia, with up to four out of five cases being linked back to Alzheimer's disease. It is an irreversible, progressive brain disorder, the sixth leading cause of death in the US, and it is estimated to affect more than 5 million Americans today, including one in nine adults age 65 and older. The number of people with the condition is expected to more than double by 2050, with someone in the US projected to develop Alzheimer's disease every 33 seconds.

For most people with Alzheimer's disease, the first symptoms appear later in life, after age 65. Scientists don't yet fully understand what causes it in older adults, especially since it may be a result of complex brain changes that happen over decades. The National Institute on Aging suggests that probable causes include a combination of genetics, environment, and lifestyle. Less than 5 percent of cases are in adults 30 to 60 years of age, and it is most often related to family history of early-onset Alzheimer's disease, though some cases appear without any known cause.

Apolipoprotein E (APOE) genotyping is a lab test that may help confirm a diagnosis of late-onset Alzheimer's disease in adults who show symptoms, but it cannot be the only tool used in diagnosis. If a person with dementia also has the APOE-e4 allele, it may be more likely that dementia is due to Alzheimer's disease, but it cannot prove it. In fact, there are no definitive diagnostic tests for Alzheimer's disease during life. This test is not appropriate for screening people without symptoms, and some people with APOE-e4 will never develop Alzheimer's disease.

Alzheimer's disease is commonly marked by memory loss, plus cognitive decline in one or more other areas, such as language skills, reasoning, attention, or visual perception. All cases of Alzheimer's disease involve cognitive decline, but not all cognitive decline is due to Alzheimer's disease.

Risk factors for late-onset Alzheimer's disease include:

- Older age

- Genetic factors (especially presence of APOE-e4)

- Family history

- History of head trauma

- Midlife hypertension

- Obesity

- Diabetes

- Hypercholesterolemia

Alzheimer's Disease and Damage to the Brain

Some researchers hypothesize that oxidative stress and inflammation—which can come from eating unhealthy food, smoking, pollution, or illness—are at the root of Alzheimer's disease. Normally, the blood-brain barrier does a good job of protecting the brain from oxidative stress and inflammation. In early Alzheimer's disease, the blood-brain barrier begins to deteriorate. This damage can be the result of inflammation.

Imagine the healthy brain is a painter's canvas on which there are smooth, uniformly colored stars (neurons) connected by orderly lines, and only clean canvas in the background. Let's use this analogy to understand five changes going on in the brain with Alzheimer's disease.

1. There is a buildup of amyloid-beta protein (also called neuritic plaques) in between neurons, like messy splotches of unwanted paint marring the clean canvas.

2. Neurofibrillary tangles (twisted fibers that block nutrition from reaching all parts of the neuron) form inside neuron cells, as if someone added excess paint to the stars, creating a raised, uneven texture.

3. Neurons die off, as if someone washed away some of the stars on the canvas.

4. There's a loss of synapses, the gap between neurons required for them to communicate. The orderly lines between stars begin to disappear. Without synapses, neurons aren't very effective.

5. The brain tissue shrinks (also known as brain atrophy), eventually affecting nearly all of its functions, as if someone put the painter's canvas in the dryer so that the resulting canvas and everything on it is a lesser version of its original.

History of Alzheimer's Disease Discovery

Alzheimer's disease is named after Dr. Alois Alzheimer. In 1906, he had a patient who died of an unusual mental illness that caused her to suffer memory loss, have language problems, and engage in unpredictable behavior. After she died, he studied her brain tissue and found two types of abnormalities. Dr. Alzheimer found the abnormal clumps we now call plaques: amyloid plaques, beta-amyloid plaques, or amyloid-beta plaques. He also found tangled bundles of fibers in the neurons, which are now called neurofibrillary tangles, fibrillary tangles, or tau tangles.

How Mental Fitness Gets Tested

Mental fitness and its decline is measured based on five areas of brain functionality, through a variety of tests. The 2015 MIND diet research used 19 standardized tests to evaluate the following five cognitive domains: episodic memory, semantic memory, perceptual speed, working memory, and visuospatial ability.

Episodic memory is a three-step process involving the ability to register personal experiences of daily events and save them as memories that can be recalled later. Think of it as the memory that stores your individual view of the events of your life, much like what a forehead camera might capture in ongoing episodes in a television series called "my life." Examples of episodic memory include recalling where you parked your car this morning, the details of your wedding day, or remembering where you were and what you were doing when you found out about the 9/11 attacks or the day JFK was assassinated.

The area of the brain important for this kind of memory is the medial temporal lobe (MTL). In the MIND diet research, it was evaluated based on results from a battery of seven tests, including: (1) word list memory, (2) word list recall, (3) word list recognition,

(4) immediate recall of a story, (5) delayed recall of a story, and (6) immediate and (7) delayed recall of a second story.

Semantic memory is the brain's reserve of general knowledge and is the kind of memory that's very useful before an exam; it's all about facts and words. Unlike episodic memory, semantic memory isn't usually connected to a specific time or place. Examples of semantic memory are the general understanding of what a key is and how it works with a door, and remembering names of colors or state capitals. It even includes remembering what a cat is and understanding how to put a sentence together. These are tidbits of information that aren't necessarily linked to a personal experience. The difference between episodic memory and semantic memory is the difference between remembering what it was like when you met your best friend and knowing that you met on a certain date. The MIND diet research measured semantic memory through three tests: (1) a naming test, (2) a verbal fluency test, and (3) an abbreviated 15-item version of the National Adult Reading Test.

Perceptual speed is the ability to examine, compare, and contrast numbers, letters, and objects quickly. It was measured in the MIND diet research by four tests: (1) a symbol-digit test that asks for certain numbers to be matched with certain geometric shapes within a short period of time, such as 90 seconds, (2) a number comparison test to measure the ability to quickly and accurately compare numbers, (3) a 30-second test of how accurately a list of color names can be read out loud when the names of the colors are printed in mismatched colors (e.g., reading the word "blue" correctly even if it's printed in red ink, and (4) a 30-second test of naming the color of the ink when mismatched with a color's name (e.g., being able to say "red" while seeing the word "blue" that is written in red ink).

Working memory is a way to temporarily store information in order to complete a mental task. It can be thought of as a form of short-term memory. In other words, it's the ability to hold on to information long enough to use it right away. It's temporary storage of information for an express purpose. For example, working memory is what helps you dial a phone number someone has just read out loud to you, or to add 14 and 73 without using a calculator, pen and paper, or any other external tools. In the MIND diet research, it was measured by three tests: (1) digit span forward, (2) digit span backward, and (3) digit ordering tests. The first two tests determine memory span by measuring the longest list of items the tested person can recite back. The lists can be of numbers, letters, or words. For the MIND diet research, numbers were used. In the first memory span test (digit span forward), the test taker had to recall the numbers in the order they were provided. In the second memory span test (digit span backward), the test taker had to remember the numbers in the reverse order that they were provided; this is a more difficult test. In addition to these two memory span tests, the third test (digit ordering test) challenged working memory ability by asking the test taker to memorize a set of numbers then recite them back in ascending order.

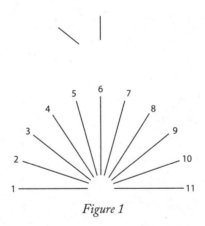

Figure 1

Visuospatial ability is the extent to which the brain can understand what it is seeing and process how it works. For example, this could include buttoning a shirt, putting together unassembled furniture, recognizing a triangle, or parking a car. It was measured by two tests: (1) a judgment of line orientation (JOLO) test, and (2) a standard progressive matrices (SPM) test. The JOLO test uses a semicircle with evenly distributed lines as the constant, then provides a series of lines in pairs. Both lines have to be accurately matched to one of the lines on the semicircle spectrum in order to pass. (See Figure 1.)

The second test, the SPM test, is a multiple-choice nonverbal test that asks the test-taker to complete a pattern or image with one of the provided options. The patterns get more difficult as the test goes on.

These 19 tests of the five cognitive domains are validated measures of cognitive function.

CHAPTER 2
The MIND Studies

What Is the MIND Diet?

The MIND diet is a healthy, evidence-based way to eat that is designed to help prevent Alzheimer's disease and delay cognitive decline. The two key MIND diet studies show how the diet keeps the aging brain seven and a half years younger and reduces the risk of developing Alzheimer's disease by 53 percent.

Researchers from Rush University Medical Center and Harvard University developed the MIND diet. The research team, led by Dr. Martha Clare Morris, director of nutritional epidemiology in the department of internal medicine at RUMC in Chicago, designed the new diet on the foundation of the Mediterranean and Dietary Approaches to Stop Hypertension (DASH) diets, modifying it based on the results from studies that specifically examined brain health. (Both the Mediterranean and DASH diets have shown promise in the area of brain health, though neither was designed for it.) The MIND diet is a selection of the most brain-healthy foods from two well-established healthy diets, supported by what we currently know from nutrition and dementia research.

MIND is an acronym for Mediterranean-DASH diet Intervention for Neurodegenerative Delay. It was ranked second only to the DASH diet as the best overall diet by *U.S. News &*

World Report's "2016 Best Diets Rankings." Top-ranked diets have to be easy to follow, nutritious, safe, effective for weight loss, and protective against diabetes and heart disease. The MIND diet does all that and hones in on the foods that specifically benefit brain health.

The MIND diet is made up of 15 components, including 10 brain-healthy food types to consume and five brain-harming ones to avoid. The healthy food groups are whole grains, vegetables in general, green, leafy vegetables, nuts, beans, berries, poultry, fish, olive oil, and wine. The harmful food groups are butter and stick margarine, whole-fat cheese, fried fast foods, red meat, and pastries and sweets.

Earning the top MIND diet score of 15 means eating at least three servings of whole grains, one serving of vegetables, and one glass of wine each day; in addition, it means eating leafy greens nearly every day (at least six times a week), nuts most days of the week (at least five times a week), beans about every other day (four times a week), berries twice a week, poultry twice a week, fish once a week, and using olive oil as the main oil. Finally, it means limiting as much as possible the foods that aren't great for brain health, but definitely consuming less than 1 tablespoon of butter or margarine a day, pastries and sweets fewer than five times a week, red meat fewer than four times a week, less than one serving of whole-fat cheese each week, and fried fast food less than once a week. Meeting each of these requirements earns one point each, adding up to a total possible score of 15.

It is worth noting that the MIND diet is less demanding than either the Mediterranean or DASH diets, with fewer required servings of fish, grains, fruits, and vegetables, and no emphasis on dairy or limits on total fat. The MIND diet is also different because it specifically recommends green, leafy vegetables as well as other vegetables, but doesn't have a fruit recommendation other than a specific recommendation for berries, such as blueberries, pomegranates, raspberries, blackberries, and strawberries.

The MIND diet's benefits to cognitive health make sense when considering the evidence-based approach to selecting its antioxidant-rich and anti-inflammatory foods, which protect the brain and make it harder for damaging plaques to form. Removing the brain-harming foods may be just as, if not more important, since eating too much of them damages the blood-brain barrier and promotes the formation of damaging beta-amyloid or amyloid-beta plaques.

One Smart Diet from Two Healthy Ones

Before there was a MIND diet, the Mediterranean and DASH diets were being studied for clues about how they affect cognitive decline, though that wasn't the focus. Since both diets have been shown to protect against high blood pressure, cardiovascular disease, stroke, and diabetes, looking at brain health was logical as those same conditions raise the risk for cognitive decline.

The Mediterranean diet is a plant-based eating pattern that emphasizes fruits, vegetables, whole grains, beans, nuts, legumes, olive oil, herbs and spices, and seafood. In moderation, it also includes poultry, eggs, cheese, yogurt, and optional wine. It limits red meat and sweets. Research has proven its benefits for heart health and diabetes.

The DASH diet is also plant based. It was designed to lower blood pressure and emphasizes grains, vegetables, fruit, low-fat or fat-free dairy, nuts, seeds, and legumes, with occasional lean meat, poultry, and fish. It limits fats, sweets, and salt. Rigorous studies show that following the DASH diet lowers blood pressure, increases beneficial HDL cholesterol, and decreases harmful LDL cholesterol and triglycerides.

The Mediterranean diet is different from the DASH diet because it uses olive oil as the main fat, is high in fish, and includes a moderate amount of wine with meals. The DASH diet is different from the Mediterranean diet in that it specifically restricts saturated fat and commercial pastries and sweets, and promotes dairy intake.

The MIND, Mediterranean, and DASH diets all share the idea of eating natural, plant-based foods and limiting animal foods and foods high in saturated fat. The MIND diet is different in that it does not specifically recommend fruit, dairy, or multiple fish meals per week. It does, however, specifically recommend berries and green, leafy vegetables.

Study 1: Cutting Alzheimer's Risk in Half

New research has found that it's possible to reduce the risk of developing Alzheimer's disease by 35 to 53 percent by following the MIND diet. The results are from a multiyear study published in 2015 in *Alzheimer's & Dementia*. They show that the more closely the MIND diet was followed, the bigger the benefits. However, even moderately following it had a significant impact. Participant diets were also mapped against Mediterranean and DASH diet eating patterns for comparison. Overall, when it came to reducing Alzheimer's disease risk, the MIND diet performed best.

The study looked at data from 923 people aged 58 to 98 years, who volunteered to take part in Rush University's Memory and Aging Project (MAP). MAP compared how well their diets matched up with MIND, Mediterranean, and DASH diets, and how much that was associated with the development of Alzheimer's disease. The MAP population lived in retirement communities or senior public housing units in the Chicago area. They were tested at least twice to ensure they did not have Alzheimer's disease at the start of the study. Over the course of four and a half years of follow-up, 144 new cases of Alzheimer's disease were diagnosed.

When it came to seeing how much the participants' diets reflected the MIND, Mediterranean, and DASH diets, there was a wide range of results, from eating habits that looked a lot like these healthy diets to eating patterns that looked nothing like them. This is helpful because it means we can see how a spectrum of diets was associated with Alzheimer's disease. After all, if everyone in the study had very similar scores, it'd be hard to know if diet made a difference. These results were split into three groups, where the top scores were most closely aligned with the healthy diets.

For the MIND diet, study participants' diets were scored based on a total possible score of 15, one point for each of the 15 MIND diet components. The top third of scores averaged 9.6 on the 15-point MIND scale, with results ranging from 8.5 to 12.5. The middle third of scores averaged 7.5 points, ranging from 7 to 8 points. Both of these groups had a significantly lower risk of developing Alzheimer's disease. The top third cut their risk by 53 percent, and the middle third cut their risk by 35 percent. For the Mediterranean diet, the top third of scores had a protective effect, cutting risk by 54 percent. Similarly, it was the top third of scores for the DASH diet that was linked to a significant risk reduction, though it was lower at 39 percent.

The researchers considered why strictly following the DASH diet was not as protective as the other two diets. They looked at what was unique to the DASH diet—that is, a specific recommendation for dairy and low salt—and suggested that perhaps these guidelines may not be particularly important for brain health. What this all means is that following any of these diets strictly will have a benefit, but that the MIND diet brings benefits even when halfway followed. Further, the MIND diet is less demanding in many ways, including fewer required servings of fish, grains, fruits, and vegetables, and no emphasis on dairy or limits on total fat.

It's tempting to wonder if the people with scores in the top third of the group were different in substantial ways. Maybe they were younger, more educated, exercised more, or took part in more brain-stimulating activities such as reading, playing games, writing letters, or visiting the library. However, the results controlled for all these factors and still found a statistically significant and clinically meaningful benefit to eating according to the MIND diet. The MIND diet was slightly less protective in people with the potential genetic marker for late-onset Alzheimer's disease, APOE-e4 (even though it's a marker, having it doesn't necessarily mean dementia is inevitable). It's important to note that the MIND diet was still protective in this group, just less so.

Another reasonable question to ask is if the results for the MIND diet were simply due to reducing the risk of diabetes, high blood pressure, stroke, and heart attack, which are all related to increased risk of Alzheimer's disease. While these factors certainly didn't hurt and were a natural benefit of a diet based on the Mediterranean and DASH diets, they were also controlled for, and the only difference was that the MIND diet was actually more protective for people who had had a heart attack in the past. Overall, the effect of the MIND diet was independent of other healthy lifestyle choices or cardiovascular-related conditions.

The study's greatest strength is its robust methodology, including good design, sampling, data collection, and data analysis. Solid methods provide assurance that results are valid and credible.

A couple of notes about the population that was studied: First, the study participants were older adults, so it's hard to extend the findings to younger adults. However, the research does suggest that those who followed the diet longer were more protected against Alzheimer's, so it's reasonable to think there is a benefit to start following the MIND diet early. Second, the study population was mostly white, making it harder to definitively extend these findings to different ethnic or racial groups. That being said, the MIND diet is a generally healthy eating pattern based on two proven diets, and a safe and nutritious choice for most people.

Study 2: Slowing Cognitive Decline

The MIND diet can slow down the effects of aging on the brain by seven and a half years, according to another multiyear study published in 2015 in *Alzheimer's & Dementia*. Over nearly five years of follow-up, the MIND diet was shown to have a big impact on slowing the cognitive decline that comes with aging for adults whose average age was about 81 years. Similar to the study on diet and risk of Alzheimer's disease, the Mediterranean and DASH diets had protective effects, but the strongest association was with the MIND diet.

The study looked at data from 960 people drawn from the more than 40 retirement communities and senior public housing units in the Chicago area that took part in Rush University's MAP. These people did not suffer from dementia at the beginning of the study and agreed to annual clinical neurological exams. However, out of 960 people, 220 had mild cognitive impairment to start. They were still included in the main analysis, though were taken out of additional secondary analysis. This is useful to see how the MIND diet can help those with mild symptoms of cognitive decline as well as those without any signs or symptoms of dementia yet. The MIND diet was found to be protective for the entire group, but even more so when the 220 were removed from the analysis, suggesting that eating for brain health before symptoms show up has bigger benefits.

The MIND diet scores for the group were divided into three tiers and compared to participant results from a battery of 19 cognitive tests that evaluated five cognitive domains: episodic memory, working memory, semantic memory, visuospatial ability, and perceptual speed. People in the top tier of MIND diet scores had higher scores across all five cognitive domains, but the diet had the strongest impact on three domains: episodic memory, semantic memory, and perceptual speed.

During the course of the study, 144 people dramatically improved or worsened how they ate. Since the dietary habits of these people changed over time, so did their MIND diet scores. To see if the inconsistent data from this portion of the group had much of an impact on the final results, the research team ran an analysis after removing this group. What they found was that doing so cleaned up the data, and the benefits of the MIND diet became even clearer and stronger. The global cognitive scores improved quite a bit as did most of the individual cognitive domains. These improved by 30 to 78 percent, with the exception of visuospatial ability, which remained stable.

To ensure these results were due to the MIND diet and not the cardiovascular protection provided by its foundation in the Mediterranean and DASH diets, the researchers controlled for high blood pressure, history of stroke or heart attack, and type 2 diabetes, but the results did not change. They also adjusted the results to account for differences in age, sex, education level, calorie intake, physical activity level, history of smoking, participation in cognitive activities, and even the genetic marker APOE-e4 that is more common in people with Alzheimer's disease. Still no appreciable effect on the beneficial results of the MIND diet. Last but not least, they took depression and obesity factors out of the picture, but adjusting for these factors also did not change any of the results. This all suggests that the MIND diet can indeed keep brains cognitively younger despite a wide range of differences.

The study has additional strengths, including its up to 10 years of follow-up, annual evaluation of cognitive function using a series of standardized tests, and validated measuring tools to assess diet, controlling for confounding factors such as physical activity and education.

Preventing cognitive decline is more important than ever since it is an identifying characteristic of dementia. Delaying cognitive decline could mean delaying dementia by years. Even those not at risk for developing Alzheimer's dementia can benefit from slowing down the normal age-related downturn in cognitive abilities. Last but not least, the MIND diet has additional benefits for heart health, diabetes, and overall nutrition and health.

CHAPTER 3
Brain-Healthy Foods

Vegetables

Vegetables, leafy greens in particular, are emphasized in the MIND diet. Past population-based studies have reported that people who best maintained their cognitive abilities ate more vegetables, especially green, leafy vegetables. Green, leafy vegetables provide folate, vitamin E, carotenoids, and flavonoids, which have been related to lower risk of dementia and cognitive decline in lab settings too.

To test the connection, researchers from Boston's Brigham and Women's Hospital and Harvard School of Public Health started looking at vegetables (and fruit) as possible protectors of cognitive health. They reduce the risk of cardiovascular disease, and cardiovascular disease is linked to an increased risk of cognitive decline. The researchers studied more than a decade's worth of diet records from 13,000 older women in search of links to cognitive performance, cognitive decline, and episodic memory in particular since this type of memory is one of the stronger predictors for Alzheimer's disease.

A serving of vegetables per day protected against cognitive decline, equal to being about one and a half years younger, cognitively speaking. Of the vegetables, the strongest protective effect was seen for green, leafy vegetables such as spinach or romaine. On average, people ate anywhere from one-third of a serving to about a serving and a half with greater benefits for higher intakes. A serving of fresh leafy greens is a cup; for cooked greens, a serving is half a cup.

Cruciferous vegetables such as broccoli and cauliflower were also clear winners for cognitive performance. The group who ate the most cruciferous vegetables, out of five groups, performed better at the cognitive tests, especially for episodic memory. Compared to the lowest intake group (who ate less than 2 tablespoons of cruciferous vegetables a day), those in the highest intake group (who ate closer to a ½-cup serving per day) performed at a level equivalent to being almost two years cognitively younger. The benefits to cognitive aging started showing up at the fourth highest intake group (eating between about ¼ cup and ½ cup of cruciferous vegetables a day). Therefore, there may be a cognitive health-related benefit to making one of your servings of daily vegetables a cruciferous one.

The researchers note that folate might be an important nutrient that could help explain the positive results for vegetables in general, as well as leafy greens and cruciferous vegetables in particular. Folate intake has been associated with cognitive function and dementia in other population-based studies. There's also a reasonable rationale for how it works. Without enough folate, levels of homocysteine can rise too high. In cell and animal studies, high homocysteine levels are toxic to neurons. The micronutrient folate is found naturally in many wholesome foods, including dark green, leafy vegetables, citrus fruits, legumes, and vegetables in general. Though it's found in both fruits and vegetables, overall, vegetables are a better source of this important nutrient.

The MIND diet includes a daily serving of any vegetable, plus a near-daily serving of leafy greens per week (six servings a week). To make it simple, consider adopting a daily green salad habit.

Some of the most commonly eaten vegetables in the United States are potatoes (much of it as fries or chips), lettuce, onions, tomatoes (much of it as pasta sauce), carrots, corn, green beans, peppers, and broccoli. These are great, but there is so much more to the vegetable world.

Generally, for quality and food safety, buy vegetables that are not bruised, slimy, or otherwise damaged. When buying precut veggies, make sure they come from a refrigerated area; if it's not refrigerated, it should be surrounded by ice. Fresh veggies should be kept separate from raw meat, poultry, and seafood in the cart, at checkout, and at home. For the convenience minded, packaged salad greens are available in prewashed ready-to-eat packages. However, adding a handling step means another opportunity to introduce food safety risks and will usually come at a premium cost, so only buy from producers you trust. Frozen vegetables are another healthy and nutritious option available all year round.

Year-Round Leafy Greens

Leafy greens hit their stride in the spring, but various greens are available in the other seasons, and some are available year round. Wash all leafy greens before consuming unless they are labeled as prewashed.

Amaranth—Not to be confused with the whole grain by the same name, this refers to the amaranth plant's leaves, not the seeds (grains). A beautiful leafy green with reddish veins, amaranth is also known as Chinese spinach, with a flavor between spinach and mild cabbage. Its stems can be prepared like asparagus, and the leaves can be treated like spinach. Choose crisp bunches with no signs of insect damage. It can be stored in a plastic bag in the refrigerator for up to a week. Amaranth is rich in vitamins A, C, and K. It provides calcium, and can be added to salads and soups alike.

Bok choy—A delicate leafy green that lends itself well to a quick steam or sauté (especially baby bok choy, which is milder than its adult version), bok choy has been grown in China for more than 6,000 years. It can also be eaten fresh. Alternate names are pak choi, bok choi, and Chinese cabbage. It's an excellent source of vitamins A and C, and a good source of folate. Look for firm stalks and fresh-looking, unwilted leaves without brown spots. Store in a plastic bag for up to a week, unwashed.

Cabbage—An affordable superfood that is high in vitamin C and low in calories, green cabbage stays fresh when refrigerated for up to a week. Keep in mind that vitamin C is destroyed through heated cooking, so a raw marinated slaw will save more of its nutrition. Look for cabbage heads that feel heavy for their size, with tight leaves.

Dandelion greens—Dandelions are technically weeds, but value is in the eye of the beholder. The greens are packed with vitamins A, C, and K, fiber, calcium, manganese, iron, and B vitamins B1, B2, and B6. The small, jagged leaves are bitter with a peppery flavor, similar to arugula. They can be used raw in a salad, tossed with a citrus vinaigrette that's vibrant enough to stand up to the bitter notes. Dandelion greens also work great mixed into soups, warm grain salads, and braised on their own.

Gai lan—Sometimes called Chinese kale or Chinese broccoli, gai lan is a dark green leafy vegetable with smoother, more tender leaves than either kale or broccoli. It's easy to enjoy this vegetable steamed or sautéed. Gai lan is an excellent source of vitamins A and C, and also provides a good source of iron and calcium. Look for fresh stalks and dark green leaves without any brown spots. Store unwashed in a plastic bag in the refrigerator for up to three days.

Salad Savoy®—This bright purple and green leafy vegetable is a child of the 1980s, developed by John Moore and grown in Salinas,

California. It's an excellent source of vitamins A, C, and fiber. Look for vibrantly colored leaves and avoid any limp or yellowing leaves. It can be stored for up to five days, unwashed, in the refrigerator, wrapped in a damp paper towel and paper bag.

Swiss chard—The leaves resemble flat kale, and its stem resembles celery. The stems can be green, red, or a rainbow mix of reds, pinks, oranges, and yellows. A hearty vegetable, Swiss chard can be used in soups, scrambles, quiche, and stir fry, or steamed. With all the varieties, some sort of Swiss chard is always in season. It's an excellent source of vitamins A and C, and also provides magnesium. Look for fresh green leaves and avoid discolored or yellowing leaves. It can be stored unwashed in plastic bags in the refrigerator crisper for two to three days.

Fall Leafy Greens

Butter lettuce—see page 39 below.
Endive—see page 41.
Ong choy spinach—see page 41.

Winter Leafy Greens

Kale—A member of the cabbage family, kale is an excellent source of vitamins A and C, and also provides calcium and potassium. There are several varieties of kale, from the common curly kale to the smoother (but still bumpy) and darker lacinato kale, also known as dinosaur kale. Kale can be stored in a plastic bag in the coldest part of the refrigerator (the bottom, back) for up to five days. Though it is a winter vegetable, its popularity has made it a year-round staple at many grocery stores.

Spring Leafy Greens

Butter lettuce—This mild, slightly sweet, and buttery lettuce is an excellent source of vitamin A, and a good source of vitamin

C and folate. Boston lettuce and Bibb lettuce are both types of butter lettuce. Look for fresh-looking leaves without signs of wilting. It can be washed, dried, and stored in a plastic bag for up to five days in the refrigerator. Sometimes butter lettuce is sold as "living lettuce" with roots still attached to dirt in order to preserve freshness. For this kind of butter lettuce, store it as-is, remove the roots, and rinse just before using.

Collard greens—Part of the cabbage family, collard greens grow in a loose bouquet and can be cooked quickly, but also stand up to slow-cooking methods like stewing and braising. These greens are an excellent source of vitamins A and C, folate, calcium, and fiber. Look for dark green leaves without yellowing. Collards can be stored in plastic bags in the refrigerator for up to five days.

Manoa lettuce—A mini lettuce with a fresh green hue that's popular in Hawaii where it's grown, manoa lettuce works great in fresh salads and can be substituted for romaine, butter, or any other salad green. Look for fresh leaves without any wilting, and store it, washed and dried, in a plastic bag in the refrigerator for up to five days. Similar to butter lettuce, manoa lettuce is sometimes sold as "living lettuce" with roots still attached to dirt. Store this kind as-is and simply separate and rinse just before using. Manoa lettuce is a vitamin A superstar and also provides vitamin C and folate.

Red leaf lettuce—Similar to romaine lettuce, red leaf lettuce is mostly green with red-tipped leaves. It's most commonly enjoyed raw in fresh salads. Red leaf lettuce is rich in vitamins A and K, and a good source of manganese. Rinse and dry leaves on paper towels before storing in plastic bags in the refrigerator for up to a week.

Sorrel—A staple of traditional Eastern European and Russian dishes, sorrel is often used as an herb in soups, sauces, and mixed into salads (but it's flavor is too strong to be the base leafy green for a salad). It has a lemony tang that is milder in the spring and more bitter by late fall. Look for green leaves with a fresh scent and avoid brown or wilted leaves. It's best used soon after purchase, but can be stored unwashed in a plastic bag in the refrigerator crisper for up to three days. Sorrel is rich in vitamins A and C, and also provides magnesium and manganese.

Spinach—The workhorse of the leafy greens, spinach deserves its healthy reputation. It's an excellent source of fiber, vitamins A and C, iron, and folate, and provides magnesium. It's been popular in the United States since the early 19th century and is enjoyed both raw in salads or as a cooked side dish. Look for fresh, crisp-looking greens with no evidence of damage from insects. Spinach can be stored in the refrigerator for up to five days, loosely wrapped in damp paper towels and in a plastic bag.

Watercress—A small leafy green that can be mixed into salads and cooked dishes (but not as the main base leafy green), watercress comes from the mustard family and adds a unique bite to any dish. It's an excellent source of vitamins A and C, and a good source of calcium. Watercress should be green without any yellowing or slippery stems, and can be stored up to five days in the refrigerator in a plastic bag after stems are cut, rinsed, and blotted with a paper towel.

Summer Leafy Greens

Butter lettuce—see page 39.

Endive—Closely related to dandelion, it too has a bite and strong enough flavor to stand up to bold vinaigrettes. Endive can be substituted for dandelion or arugula in recipes. It is fiber-rich and provides vitamin C, calcium, iron, phosphorus, and potassium. Look for crisp and bright green leaves and avoid wilted or browning leaves. It can be stored for up to a week in the refrigerator.

Manoa lettuce—see page 40.

Ong choy spinach—A tropics- and subtropics-loving green, ong choy is also called river spinach or water spinach because it is grown in water. It's popular in Southeast Asian dishes and is commonly used in stir-fry dishes. It looks like a smaller, flatter-leaf spinach, and is an excellent source of iron, vitamins A and C, and a good source of calcium. Look for moist green leaves and stay away from dark, dry, or bruised leaves. Stems should be crisp and green. It's commonly found in Asian markets. Ong choy spinach can be wrapped with damp paper towels and stored in an airtight container in the refrigerator for one to two days.

Year-Round Vegetables—Beyond Leafy Greens

Bell peppers—Whether red, yellow, or green, bell peppers should be heavy for their size with brightly colored tight skin. They can be stored in a plastic bag in the refrigerator for up to five days. Low in calories and high in water and vitamin C, bell peppers are perfect for crudités or stir fries.

Broccoflower—As one would imagine, this is a cross between broccoli and cauliflower, and looks a bit like green cauliflower. The head should be firm and compact without any brown spots or wilted leaves. It's rich in vitamin C, and provides folate and fiber too. Store refrigerated for up to five days. Enjoy raw, braised, roasted, or sautéed.

Broccolini—Sweeter than broccoli due to the cross-breeding with gai lan (see page 38), broccolini stalks are soft and edible. Rich in vitamins A and C, broccolini can be refrigerated in a plastic bag, unwashed, for a week and a half. Its delicate, sweet flavor does well simply steamed or with a quick sauté.

Carrots—These can be orange, purple, white, red, or yellow. Look for smooth, firm, crisp carrots with deep color and fresh green tops. Avoid soft, wilted, or split carrots. Rich in vitamins A and C.

Celeriac—Also known as celery root, celeriac is rough and knobby with an uneven surface and mottled brown-white outer layer. Peel the outer layer away to expose a creamy white interior that can be chopped up and used like potatoes—in home fries, roasted, or pureed into soups. It can also be made into a mash, or the raw form can be sliced thin for slaws and salads. Store in the refrigerator for up to a week. It's rich in vitamins C and K, and a good source of fiber and potassium.

Celery—An underrated vegetable, celery offers a satisfying, crisp crunch along with vitamins A and C. Look for straight, rigid stalks with fresh leaves. Refrigerate for up to a week or more. Try celery stalks with French mustard for a simple snack.

Cherry tomatoes—Store at room temperature away from direct sunlight and enjoy within a week after ripening; they taste best unrefrigerated. Rich in vitamins A and C, cherry tomatoes also provide vitamin K and potassium. Versatile, they can be tossed into pasta sauces, soups, and salads, or enjoyed raw for a snack.

Chinese eggplant—Purple and the shape of a small zucchini, Chinese eggplant is sweeter and more tender than conventional eggplant. It can be cooked without peeling or salting, so you get the benefit of the polyphenols in the skin. Look for eggplant that is heavy for its size with firm, glossy skin. Refrigerate and use within a week.

Leeks—Related to onions, leeks have a nuanced, sweeter flavor. They look like large green onions with white bulbs and green tops. Leeks are rich in vitamin A and a good source of folate and vitamin C. Store them unwashed in a plastic bag for up to two weeks. Thinly slice the white bulb to add to savory dishes, and slice the green tops for garnish.

Mushrooms—Rich in a satisfying umami flavor, mushrooms make a nutritious and flavorful meat alternative. They're low in calories, a good source of B vitamins, and contain some vitamin D. Look for mushrooms that are firm, without spots or slime.

Onions—Offering immense flavor without the salt, onions are an unsung hero of delicious dishes. They're also high in vitamin C and a good source of fiber. Onions should be stored similar to potatoes, in a cool, dark, well-ventilated place for up to four weeks. Cut onions can be stored in the refrigerator for use within two to three days.

Parsnips—Pale white and shaped like large carrots, parsnips should be firm and dry, and without pits. Look for smaller ones for a flavorful and more tender treat. A good source of vitamin C, folate, and fiber, parsnips' sugar develops with cold weather, so though they are available year-round, try them in the late fall, after a frost. Store in the produce drawer for two to three weeks.

Pearl onions—About the size of a large marble and commonly eaten whole, pearl onions are otherwise like regular onions and come in white, yellow, and red varieties, and pack flavor and vitamin C. Look for onions that are dry, with papery skins still attached.

Potatoes—High in vitamin C and potassium. Look for potatoes that are clean, firm, smooth, dry, and uniform in size. They can be stored in a cool, dry, well-ventilated place for three to five weeks. Starchy russets are best for mashing, and waxy Yukon Gold, red, white, and fingerling potatoes are better for roasting. Purple potatoes are great for steaming or baking.

Snow peas—Shiny and flat, with small peas in the pod, snow peas should be stored unwashed in a perforated bag in the refrigerator for up to a week. They are mild and slightly sweet, and can be enjoyed raw, steamed, stir fried, or mixed into salads or pasta dishes.

Yucca root—Brown on the outside, white on the inside, vitamin C–rich yucca root can be used in soups in place of potatoes. Store in a cool, dark, dry place for up to a week, or peel, wrap tightly, and store in the freezer for several months.

Fall Vegetables

Acorn squash—Shaped like an acorn, it even has a mildly nutty flavor. The skin should be dull, without any soft spots or cracks. As with other squash, look for something heavy for its size. Store away from extreme temperatures and sunlight, in a cool, dry area. It can stay fresh for up to three months. It's a good source of vitamin C and only 30 calories per half cup.

Black salsify—Also known as an oyster plant because of the root's oyster-like flavor. Meanwhile, the leaves, if attached, can be used as a salad green. The long root should have a black skin and creamy interior. Look for smooth and firm roots. Cut off the root end, peel off the outer skin, spritz with lemon juice to keep it from browning, cube it and add to soups, or boil and mash like potatoes. Avoid overcooking, as it can become stringy and mushy.

Broccoli—Super nutritious, broccoli is rich in vitamin C and folate, and a good source of fiber and potassium. The heads should be tight and florets should be bluish-green. Refrigerate and use within three to five days.

Brussels sprouts—They look like little baby cabbages and are a related vegetable. These little cruciferous vegetables are low in calories and high in vitamin C, folate, fiber, and so much more. Look for firm, compact, bright green Brussels sprouts, on the stalk if possible. Simply toss with extra-virgin olive oil, vinegar, salt, and pepper, and roast for a delicious side dish. They last refrigerated for up to a week.

Buttercup squash—A sweet, creamy orange squash, the skin of buttercup squash is dark green. Look for a squash that is heavy for its size with an even color. They can be stored in a cool, dry place for up to three months.

Butternut squash—With flesh that is a vibrant orange like pumpkin, butternut squash can be used in any recipe that calls for pumpkin. Store in a cool, dark place for up to a month. It's an excellent source of vitamins A and C, and a good source of fiber, potassium, and magnesium.

Cardoon—With a flavor that's like a blend of artichokes and celery, cardoon looks like oversized celery. A good source of potassium, magnesium, and folate, cardoon can be enjoyed cooked or raw in salads.

Cauliflower—High in vitamin C and a good source of folate, cauliflower should have compact, white curds and bright green, firmly attached leaves. Avoid brown spots or loose sections. Refrigerate in a plastic bag for up to five days. Enjoy it roasted or experiment with cauliflower "mashed potatoes" or "rice."

Chayote squash—Use anywhere summer squash would be a good fit.

Chinese long beans—These can measure up to 3 feet long, with a taste similar to green beans, and can be prepared in similar ways. However, they are more flexible (less crisp). Refrigerate in a plastic bag for up to five days. They're rich in iron, fiber, folate, potassium, and zinc. They're also a source of calcium.

Delicata squash—Also known as the peanut squash and Bohemian squash, it is an elongated squash that should appear light yellow with green striations when ripe, and light green when unripe. Rich in vitamin A. Look for squash that is heavy for its size. Delicata squash hold their shape when cooked, making them perfect for stuffing with whole grains, lean poultry, and vegetables.

Daikon radish—Long, white, and slender, the daikon radish should be shiny, firm, and smooth. It's low in calories and a good source of vitamin C. Store it tightly wrapped in plastic in the refrigerator for up to three days. With a mild peppery bite, they can be used in any recipe that calls for radishes.

Garlic—So much flavor comes out of these small, white bulbs, and their sulfuric compounds are being studied for a variety of health benefits. Store in a cool, dark place, outside the refrigerator, for several weeks. Try chopping off the top of a whole bulb and roasting with extra-virgin olive oil, wrapped up in foil, until the cloves become soft, mild in flavor, and spreadable.

Ginger—A flavorful root, ginger is simply amazing and adds depth of flavor and aromatics to any dish. Look for firm roots with smooth skin and a spicy aroma. Avoid cracked or withered ginger. A good source of vitamin C, magnesium, potassium, and plenty of polyphenols, ginger can be peeled and chopped then added to stir-fry dishes, pasta sauces, smoothies, and even turkey patties.

Hearts of palm—Harvested from the central core of palm trees, they are soft and firm at the same time and offer a mildly sweet taste. They are available fresh, but are more commonly found canned or jarred, and work well sliced into salads or pureed into soups and sauces. If fresh, refrigerate immediately in a tightly sealed container for up to two weeks. Packaged hearts of palm should be stored away from direct sunlight and will stay fresh for about a week after opening. Hearts of palm are rich in potassium, vitamin C, iron, copper, zinc, and B vitamins.

Jerusalem artichokes—Looking nothing like an artichoke and related to sunflowers, which is why they are also known as sunchokes, Jerusalem artichokes are starchy tubers like potatoes or turnips. Look for firm, relatively smooth skin, and store in a plastic bag in the refrigerator for up to a week. They're a good source of iron. When roasted, the skin gets flaky and the flesh tender. The taste is slightly nutty and sweet.

Pumpkin—Indigenous to North America, pumpkins aren't just for Halloween decor. They're an excellent source of vitamin A and a good source of vitamin C. Look for pumpkins that are heavy for their size, and store in a cool, dark place for up to two months. Roast, cube, and add to salads, or roast, puree, and add to smoothies, muffins, and breads.

Sweet potatoes—A truly misunderstood vegetable, they're not actually related to potatoes and sometimes mislabeled as yams. High in vitamins A and C and a good source of potassium, sweet potatoes should be stored in a cool, dark place for up to three to five weeks. Bake, roast, or steam them, and use them in salads, puree them into pancakes, or enjoy them on their own.

Turnips—Though they come in all shapes and colors, you're most likely to see the purple and white variety. Look for heavy turnips, and keep in mind that the smaller ones are sweeter. They can be eaten raw or cooked and are rich in vitamin C. They can be stored in the refrigerator for a few days, but they get bitter with longer storage.

Winter Vegetables

Brussels sprouts—see page 45.
Buttercup squash—see page 45.
Cardoon—see page 45.
Delicata squash—see page 46.
Sweet potatoes—see page 47.
Turnips—see page 48.

Spring Vegetables

Artichokes—Choose plump, tight artichokes that are heavy for their size. They're a good source of vitamin C, fiber, folate, and magnesium. Store them refrigerated for up to a week and keep dry. Don't toss the stem—that's where the tender and delicious heart extends.

Asparagus—Available in green, purple, and white, but the green variety is often the most tender. The slimmer the stalk, the more delicate the flavor. Look for firm stalks with tight tips, and stay away from any that are limp or wilted. Wrap the ends of the stalks in a wet paper towel, and store in a plastic bag, refrigerated, for up to four days. Diagonally sliced, 1-inch pieces of asparagus, lightly sautéed, are a gorgeous and healthy add-in to warm grain salads.

Chayote squash—see page 46.

Fennel—Sometimes called sweet anise, fennel has a delicate licorice aroma and flavor. Their feathery tops can be used like an herb, and the firm white bulbs can be sliced into salads, made into slaw, sautéed, or roasted with extra-virgin olive oil. Keep it refrigerated and use within five days. Fennel is a good source of vitamin C, potassium, and fiber.

Fiddlehead ferns—So named as they resembles the curved decorative end of a fiddle, the season for this spring green is short, but worth staying vigilant for. Look for a tight coil with only an inch or two uncoiled, bright color, and firmness. Best to enjoy them as soon as possible, but they should last in the refrigerator, wrapped to avoid drying out, for up to three days. They can be prepared similarly to asparagus. Simple methods are best so that their seasonal flavor can shine through.

Green beans—Also known as string beans, green beans can be eaten fresh or cooked. Look for green beans with good color that are firm enough that they would snap easily when bent. Refrigerate and use within a week. They're a good source of vitamin C and fiber.

Morel mushrooms—A springtime darling, morel mushroom caps look like honeycombs. They should smell fresh and earthy, without soft spots, bruising, or slime. Store them, unwashed, in a paper bag in the refrigerator for up to three days. They're an excellent source of vitamin D.

Peas—Also known as sweet peas or English peas, they can be enjoyed raw or cooked. They should be firm, bright green, and medium in size. They can be refrigerated in a perforated plastic bag for three to five days. Shell just before using. Peas are a good source of vitamin A, folate, and fiber.

Vidalia onions—Georgia's official state vegetable, the Vidalia onion is sweet and savory all at the same time. They're sweet due to lower sulfur in the Georgia soil they're grown in. They can be enjoyed raw in salads, roasted, grilled, or caramelized. Like other onions, they're a good source of vitamin C.

Summer Vegetables

Armenian cucumber—About 12 to 15 inches long and pale green, this cuke is actually a melon with a mild cucumber taste. It requires no deseeding or peeling, and can be used raw in drinks, appetizers, salads, and snacks, or cooked like zucchini. A good source of water and vitamin C, store them in the refrigerator crisper for a few days.

Beets—They can't be beat. Look for firm, smooth-skinned beets, and know that the smaller they are in size, the more tender they'll be. An excellent source of folate and polyphenols, beets have an earthy, sweet flavor. They can be boiled or roasted, and the greens can be enjoyed raw or sautéed. Store in a plastic bag, refrigerated, for up to three weeks.

Chinese long beans—see page 46.

Corn—There's nothing like fresh, sweet summer corn. Look for green husks, fresh silks, and tight rows of kernels. Refrigerate with husks on and use as soon as possible, within one to two days. An easy way to prepare corn is to steam or boil it until it simply smells like corn. Corn is a good source of vitamin C.

Crookneck squash—A vitamin C–rich yellow summer squash that is quick cooking, crookneck squash is best when no bigger than 8 inches around. Like other squashes, choose one that is heavy for its size. Refrigerate for up to a week.

Cucumbers—Crisp and mildly sweet, cucumbers should be firm, evenly shaped, and dark green in color. Look for cucumbers that are heavy for their size, and store them refrigerated, bagged, for up to a week. Cucumbers are a good source of vitamin C, are water-packed, and have natural cooling agents. Enjoy them raw as a simple snack, in salads, in cucumber sandwiches, or scoop out the seeds to make cucumber cups and fill with hummus for an easy appetizer.

Eggplant—Look for eggplants that are heavy for their size, without discoloration. They can be stored in the crisper for five to seven days. Due to their meaty and toothsome texture, eggplants are a popular center-of-plate item for plant-based eaters. They soak up flavor like a sponge.

French beans—Similar to but slimmer than green beans, they are also known as haricots verts. French beans should be bright in color and crisp. Store them in a plastic bag, refrigerated, for one to two weeks. They're an excellent source of fiber, B vitamins, folate, magnesium, and potassium. Try them blanched and added to salads, alongside ahi tuna steaks, or in an Asian stir-fry dish.

Garlic—see page 46.

Grape tomatoes—see cherry tomatoes on page 43.

Green beans—see page 49.

Hearts of palm—see page 47.

Okra—Slippery when cooked, okra tastes great paired with tomatoes in stews. Look for firm, brightly colored pods and refrigerate for up to three days. Okra is an excellent source of vitamin C, and a good source of folate and fiber.

Peas—see page 49.

Radishes—Rich in vitamin C, radishes are crisp and peppery, adding a bright note to any salad or savory dish. Tops should be green and fresh, roots should be smooth and bright. They can be refrigerated in a plastic bag for use within a week.

Shallots—Related to onions, but more delicate, sweet, and mild, shallots should be firm and heavy for their size, with dry, papery skins. They can be stored in a cool, dark, well-ventilated place for up to four weeks. Cut shallots should be refrigerated, tightly sealed, and used within two to three days. They are a good source of vitamins A and C.

Sugar snap peas—Enjoy as soon as possible to get a sweet, crisp taste, which diminishes with storage time. They can be kept in the crisper in a perforated plastic bag for up to two days. Sugar snap peas are rich in vitamin C and a good source of vitamin K. Simply pull back the fibrous seam and enjoy them as a fresh snack.

Tomatillos—Also known as tomate verde and Mexican husk tomato, the tomatillo is a small, green tomato surrounded by a papery husk. Look for dry, hard tomatillos with tight husks. They can be refrigerated in the crisper for two to three weeks. An excellent source of vitamin C, one of the easiest and tastiest ways to enjoy them is in salsas. Simply peel away the papery skin, and puree with onions, peppers, cilantro, and a pinch of salt.

Tomatoes—Look for bright, shiny skins and firm flesh, and store away from direct sunlight. They should be enjoyed within a week after ripening and taste best when not refrigerated. They are rich in vitamins A and C, and provide lycopene and potassium.

Yukon Gold potatoes—A cross between the North American white potato and a wild South American yellow potato, Yukons are rich in vitamin C and a good source of potassium. Store them in a cool, dark, well-ventilated place and use within three to five weeks. They are waxy with a firm texture, making them great for roasting, soups, stews, and gratins because they keep their shape.

Zucchini—A summer squash, zucchini skin should be firm, slightly prickly, shiny, and free from cuts or bruises. Zucchini can be stored in the refrigerator, in a plastic bag, for four to five days. It is high in vitamin C and quick cooking, making it ideal for a stir fry, chopped into an omelet, added to casseroles and sauces, or simply grilled.

Whole Grains

Whole grains are an important part of the daily diet in the MIND, Mediterranean, and DASH diets. Whole grains are a kind of seed. To be considered whole, a grain must contain all of the essential parts and naturally occurring nutrition of the entire seed or kernel, including all of the germ seed, fleshy endosperm, and outer bran.

Whole grains provide an excellent source of vitamin E, which has been proven to protect the brain.

New evidence suggests whole grains have always played a key role in brain health, starting as early as millions of years ago. Researchers in Europe and Australia studied the role of diet with early humans, noting that carbs from whole grains, roots, and starchy plant foods were required to support the increased metabolic demands of a growing brain. While many people associate early humans with meat-based diets, it was actually cooked starches that helped accelerate brain size starting in the Middle Pleistocene time.

Today, whole grains are being studied for benefits for cardiovascular disease, diabetes, cancers, cognitive health, and more. According to the Whole Grains Council, "because of the phytochemicals and antioxidants, people who eat three daily servings of whole grains have been shown to reduce their risk of heart disease by 25 to 36 percent, stroke by 37 percent, type 2 diabetes by 21 to 27 percent, digestive system cancers by 21 to 43 percent, and hormone-related cancers by 10 to 40 percent."

Cognitive benefits of eating whole grains may start early. In a 2015 study, elementary school students scored higher in all areas of testing after eating breakfast. Those who ate more whole grains had significantly higher scores in reading comprehension, verbal fluency, and math. Whole grains also play a role in neuroprotection later in life.

One study of more than 2,000 older Swedish adults suggests that neuroprotective diets should include whole grains, vegetables, nuts, legumes, and fish, while unhealthy diets included foods such as refined grains, processed foods, red meat, and sugar. Another study found that the anti-inflammatory protection provided by whole grains slowed cognitive decline among more than 5,000 middle-aged adults. Not surprisingly, the highest levels of inflammation were linked to diets high in red meat and fried food, and lower in whole grains. The bottom line is that overall diet patterns higher in whole grains are shown to slow cognitive decline.

Cooking grains is a simple proposition, and the main downside is the time it takes. A little preplanning can take care of this. However, for the days when you need whole grains in a hurry, there are high-quality frozen and 10-minute par-cooked whole grains on the market with little to no nutritional compromise. From ancient grains to modern quick-cooking versions, whole grains have a lot to offer.

Amaranth—A small, gluten-free, ancient pseudo-grain, amaranth is higher in protein than most other grains at 14 percent, and contains lysine, an amino acid not commonly found in grains. It has a nutty, peppery flavor and a crunchy texture at its center, even when fully cooked, making it ideal for adding to salads and baked goods. Amaranth is most often if not always sold in whole grain form. Prepare 6 cups of water to 1 cup of dry amaranth, then drain. A half-cup, cooked serving is a good source of iron and magnesium.

Barley—A fiber superstar, barley is 17 to 30 percent fiber (by comparison, whole wheat is 12 percent fiber, oats are 10 percent fiber, and corn is 7 percent fiber). Generally, a grain's fiber is in its outer bran layer. Interestingly, in barley, fiber is found throughout the grain, so even refined barley will have some fiber. Still, look for whole grain barley labeled with terms such as "whole barley," "dehulled barley," "hulled barley," or "hull-less barley," and bypass the refined versions that may be labeled as "pearled" or "quick-cooking" barley.

Buckwheat—Previously known as a poor man's food, it grows well on rocky hillsides and is hardy enough to thrive without pesticides. Today it enjoys health food chic and has gotten attention for containing the antioxidant rutin, which may improve circulation. Like amaranth, buckwheat is not a true grain and is not even wheat, despite its name. In fact, unlike all true wheat varieties, buckwheat is gluten-free. Japanese soba noodles are traditionally made with buckwheat; it is also used in crepes.

Bulgur—When wheat kernels have been boiled, dried, and cracked, the result is bulgur. Because it has already been precooked and dried, prepare it like dry pasta because it's ready after about 10 minutes of boiling. It's commonly used in a dish called tabbouleh, a grain salad with bulgur, mint, parsley, tomatoes, extra-virgin olive oil, and lemon juice. Bulgur provides more fiber than quinoa, oats, millet, buckwheat, or corn.

Corn—More commonly thought of as a movie theater snack or summer picnic vegetable, corn is still in fact a whole grain. DNA testing shows corn originally came from Mexico, where it was developed into an agricultural staple about 9,000 years ago. Corn is a gluten-free grain that provides more vitamin A and related carotenoids than most other grains.

It gets a bad rap as most of the corn in the US and Canada is used to feed animals (called dent or field corn), but there are other unique varieties that have a role in human diets. Sweet corn is the kind that is in season in the summer and can be eaten off the cob. It should be eaten soon after harvesting because the sugars start converting to starches as soon as it's picked. If you need to store it, leave it in the husk.

When eaten with beans, corn helps provide complete proteins. In traditional Central and South American culinary cultures, corn is commonly soaked in lime water, which adds calcium and increases B-vitamin absorption. Corn products that commonly go through this process are masa flour, tortillas, and the southern US's hominy.

Einkorn—An ancient wheat variety that fell out of favor as a mainstream crop because of how difficult it is to remove its hull, einkorn is still grown in some areas of Europe, and more recently has had a resurgence in Washington state. Einkorn is a drought-tolerant grain that is just about always in whole grain form. Among wheat varieties, it has the highest levels of carotenoids such as lutein, zeaxanthin, and beta-carotene. Though it still contains gluten and the wheat protein gliadin, einkorn is less allergenic compared to other types of wheat.

Farro (aka Emmer)—Farro, as it's known in Italy, is another ancient wheat variety and was one of the first domesticated grains grown in the Fertile Crescent in the Middle East (modern-day Iraq, Syria, Lebanon, Jordan, Israel, and Egypt). It has higher total antioxidant activity than other wheats. Similar to einkorn, farro is harder to hull than modern durum wheat, which is why it fell out of favor. Farro comes pearled (i.e., refined) and in whole grain forms, so be sure to choose whole grain farro. There are quick-cooking whole grain farro options on the market.

Freekeh—Yet another kind of wheat, freekeh is also known as farik and frikeh, and is often sold cracked into smaller quick-cooking pieces the way bulgur wheat is. Freekeh is usually made from hard durum wheat, harvested when still young and green, then roasted and rubbed. Freekeh has a smoky flavor, and works well in Middle Eastern and North African cuisine, including pilafs, grain salads, and porridges. It is commonly sold in whole grain form.

Khorasan wheat—This is an ancient wheat variety whose name comes from the ancient Egyptian name for wheat, and is about two to three times the size of most wheats. It has enjoyed a recent return to the US food supply and is most frequently sold as Kamut. It has a nutty taste and is higher in protein than other wheat because it has never been hybridized. Look for whole Kamut to make sure you're getting whole grains. It can be found whole or as flour in natural food stores, and is also in some commercial products such as pasta, puffed cereal, and crackers.

Kaniwa—This tiny pseudo-grain is cousins with quinoa (page 58). Like quinoa, kaniwa (alternatively spelled qaniwa, canihua, and canahua) is high in protein. It comes from the cold mountains of Peru and Bolivia. Unlike quinoa, kaniwa doesn't need to be rinsed as thoroughly as it's not coated with the bitter substances that need to be washed off of quinoa (called saponins). It's labor-intensive to harvest and is traditionally lightly roasted and ground into a flour before being consumed in hot and cold drinks, and porridges. Since it's a specialty item, it will most likely be sold in whole grain form, whether the word "whole" is used on the label or not. Kaniwa is gluten-free.

Millet—Millet isn't just one grain. Millet includes a group of related grains from around the world. Other names for millet are pearl millet, foxtail millet, proso millet (also called hog, common, or broom corn millet), finger millet (also called ragi), and fonio. Millet is common in India, China, South America, Russia, and the Himalayas. Millet comes in white, gray, yellow, or red varieties, and is just about always in whole grain form. India is the world's largest millet producer, where it is used to make roti, a common flatbread. It can also be used in pilafs, breakfast porridges, added to breads and soups, or popped like popcorn. It's gluten-free and high in magnesium and antioxidants.

Oats—Oats need no introduction, as just about everyone in the United States has encountered oatmeal for breakfast at one time or another. Though oats are processed in a variety of ways, their bran and germ aren't typically removed, so just about all oats on the market are in whole grain form. Most are steamed and flattened into soft, quick-cooking oats, also known as "old-fashioned," "regular," or "rolled" oats. These are the kind of oats found in instant oatmeal. For a nuttier flavor and more toothsome texture, try steel cut oats, which are sometimes called Irish or Scottish oats. To get to steel cut oats, the entire oat (which looks like a grain of rice) is sliced a couple times into smaller pieces for quicker (but not instant) cooking that takes about 20 minutes. Steel cut oatmeal is an entirely different experience compared to rolled oats.

Oats contain a soluble fiber called beta-glucan that helps lower cholesterol. They also contain antioxidants that may help protect blood vessels from LDL cholesterol damage. They can be enjoyed as the traditional breakfast porridge, in a pilaf dinner side dish, mixed into turkey burgers, or as a crispy coating for baked chicken.

Quinoa—An ancient Incan pseudo-grain from the Andes mountains, quinoa provides a complete protein and cooks in about 10 to 12 minutes, making it a convenient and super-nutritious vegetarian protein choice. It keeps its texture well, so it works great in pilafs, soups, and salads. It is a very small, round grain that has a little "tail" that pops out when it's finished cooking. Most quinoa must be rinsed before cooking to wash away bitter residue from compounds called saponins. Quinoa comes in many colors, including red, purple, orange, green, black, and yellow.

Rice—Whole grain rice is usually brown but can also be black, purple, or red, and comes in long-, medium-, or short-grain forms. The top rice-growing states in the United States are Arkansas, California, Louisiana, Mississippi, Missouri, and Texas, where rice-friendly warm, humid climates are available. Rice cookers are extremely convenient. Simply measure out the rice and water, press cook, and you're done. Make a large batch of whole grain rice and enjoy over a couple days. Rice is naturally gluten-free.

Rye—Related to wheat and long considered to be a weed, rye became valued for its ability to grow quickly and in climates too wet, cold, or drought-affected for other grains. It is a traditional staple in Northern Europe, Russia, Poland, Canada, Argentina, China, and Turkey. Look for whole rye or rye berries to ensure it is a whole grain. Rye contains a high level of fiber in both its bran and its inner endosperm, and is most commonly enjoyed as bread or crisp bread, but can also be used in soups and grain salads.

Sorghum—Also known as milo, guinea corn, Kaffir corn, durra, mtama, jowar, and kaoliang, sorghum is an ancient grain that grows well in the Great Plains, from South Dakota to Texas. Nearly always sold in its whole grain form whether it's labeled "whole" or not, sorghum is gluten-free and grown from traditional seeds, so it's naturally non-GMO. Most of the sorghum in the United States goes to animal feed or made into biodegradable packing materials. However, it can be eaten as a porridge or popped like popcorn.

Spelt—A higher-protein variety of wheat, spelt can replace wheat in most recipes. In Italy it is known as farro grande (that is, big farro). Spelt is sold in both whole and refined form, so be sure to look for whole spelt.

Teff—A tiny-sized grain that is common in Ethiopia, it is used to make the spongy, pleasantly sour flatbread called injera. Teff is a kind of millet and grows in red, purple, gray, yellowy brown, and ivory colors. It grows well in both flood and drought conditions, from sea level to mile-high altitudes. Teff is higher in calcium and resistant starch (a newly discovered type of dietary fiber) than other grains. In fact, a cup of cooked teff has about the same amount of calcium as a half cup of cooked spinach. It can be enjoyed in porridges, polenta, crepes, and breads. It cooks quickly, offers a mild flavor, and is gluten-free. It is almost always sold in whole grain form.

Triticale—Compared to all the ancient grains available, the wheat-rye hybrid triticale is a baby. Commercially grown triticale has only been around for a few decades. Rye and wheat easily cross-breed in nature, and the resulting triticale grows well without industrial fertilizers and pesticides, which makes it a good option for organic farmers. As a blend of both rye and wheat, triticale contains gluten.

Wheat—While gluten is harmful to people who are allergic to it, gluten is also the reason wheat became so valuable to bread bakers since it helps them create toothsome risen breads. There are two main varieties of wheat—hard winter durum wheat (used commonly for pasta) and soft spring bread wheat (used most often for most other wheat foods). Hard wheat has more protein and more gluten than spring wheat, making it ideal for bread baking. Soft wheat creates cake flour. It also comes in red and white varieties that refer to their color, not whether they're whole grain or not, which means it's possible to have whole white wheat made from whole grain soft white wheat. To be sure you're getting a whole grain, look for the word "whole" on the label. Wheat varieties and hybrids include wheat berries, bulgur, farro, einkorn, spelt, Kamut, durum, red wheat, white wheat, spring wheat, winter wheat, and triticale.

Wild rice—Not technically rice, it is native to the Americas and was originally grown around the Great Lakes. Today, most wild rice is still harvested by Native Americans in the Minnesota area, though it's also grown and harvested to a lesser extent in California and elsewhere in the Midwest. Wild rice has a pleasantly strong nutty flavor and firm texture, with twice the protein and fiber of brown rice (but less iron and calcium). Wild rice is just about always sold as a whole grain, and is a good source of fiber, folate, magnesium, zinc, vitamin B6, and niacin. It works great in stuffed mushrooms, grain salads, and soups, and can be popped like popcorn.

What Are Sprouted Whole Grains?

Grains used to sprout accidentally, but most grains today no longer do so by happenstance. There may be some nutritional benefits to sprouting a grain, which has led some food producers and home experimenters to purposefully sprout their grains.

The germ of a whole grain is the plant embryo, and it feeds on the starchy endosperm and bran of a whole grain until it's ready to germinate into a new plant. When temperature and moisture conditions are just right, the whole grain will sprout. When sprouting starts, enzymes make the endosperm starch easier for the germ to digest; some people may also find this "activated" type of grain easier to digest as well.

When a grain is properly and safely sprouted, it's both seed and new plant, which makes it more digestible and higher in vitamins and minerals such as B vitamins, vitamin C, folate, fiber, and an amino acid often lacking in grains, lysine.

Keep in mind that the process requires precision in the time, temperature, and moisture used. Too much moisture and the grain drowns and opens from swelling versus sprouting, and can ferment or even rot. Left for too long, a healthy sprout can continue to grow into a new grass stalk, which is not very digestible to humans.

If interested in sprouted grains, look for a brand you trust to sprout their grains under carefully controlled conditions. Remember, sprouted or not, whole grains are an extremely healthy food choice.

Nuts

The MIND diet recommends eating nuts most days (at least five times a week), in part because nuts are a rich source of vitamin E, a nutrient that protects the brain. Nuts also have a clear and well-established role in heart health. In 2003, the FDA approved the following claim: "Scientific evidence suggests but does not prove that eating 1½ ounces per day of most nuts as part of a diet low in saturated fat and cholesterol may reduce the risk of heart disease." Previous and ongoing research shows that nuts are protective for diabetes, cancers, longevity, and cognitive health.

A 2013 randomized clinical trial in Spain, called PREDIMED-NAVARRA, showed that following a Mediterranean diet with either extra nuts or olive oil resulted in higher cognitive scores compared to low-fat diets. The study participants included 522 men and women at high risk for cardiovascular disease who were on average 75 years of age. After six and a half years of being on either a Mediterranean diet with additional olive oil, or a Mediterranean diet with additional nuts, participants had significantly higher global cognitive scores compared to the low-fat control diet.

How do nuts slow down cognitive decline? To find out, the USDA reviewed several studies focusing on almonds, pecans, pistachios, and walnuts, and found that these tree nuts slow down age-related cognitive decline, perhaps because they reduce oxidative stress and inflammation. Nuts are nutrient-dense and contain a variety of bioactive compounds, including polyunsaturated fats, phytochemicals, and polyphenols. In addition to vitamin E, they provide folate, fiber, and flavonoids, such as proanthocyanidins.

In addition to cognitive health, nuts have a role in overall health and longevity. Harvard researchers examining decades of data from more than 76,000 women and more than 42,000 men in the United States found that the more nuts people ate, the longer they lived. Compared to people who didn't eat nuts, people who ate nuts seven or more times per week had a 20 percent lower death rate from heart disease, cancer, and respiratory diseases. These findings are supported by earlier studies finding longevity benefits for whites, blacks, and elderly people at five servings of nuts per week, and at three servings per week for Spanish adults at risk for heart disease.

Should you be worried about nuts and weight gain? The short answer is no. Eating nuts more often is associated with less weight gain, reduced belly fat, and a lower risk for obesity. That being said, food choices should always fit within appropriate calorie ranges.

Eating nuts at least five times a week works out nicely for a daily work-week snack habit. Nuts are antioxidant-rich nuggets of good health, and very versatile in the kitchen. They can be added to vegetable dishes, morning oatmeal, chopped and used to crust fish, in salads and stir-fry dishes, in salad dressings, or simply on their own as a healthy snack.

When selecting in-shell nuts, they should feel heavy for their size. Avoid nuts with signs of insect or moisture damage, or that rattle when shaken, which is a sign they have dried out and are old. Shells should not have holes, and most should not have cracks (the big exception is the pistachio, whose shell partially opens during the natural ripening process).

For packages of shelled nuts (kernels), look for expiration dates, avoid nuts that look rubbery or shriveled, and smell them to make sure they're not rancid. Store nuts in an airtight container in a cool dry place. They can also be refrigerated or frozen.

All nuts provide healthy unsaturated fats, and for the most part there is a good ratio of more unsaturated to less saturated fat. Some nuts contain more saturated fat than others. The easiest way to ensure you're not going overboard on saturated fat is to simply mix it up and eat a variety of nuts.

The following nuts contain a higher percentage of healthy unsaturated fats, and less than 2 grams of saturated fat per 1-ounce serving: almonds, hazelnuts, pine nuts, pistachios, and walnuts.

Healthy Nuts

Almonds—California's Central Valley grows 80 percent of the world's almond supply, and at 23 almonds per serving, whole almonds are a satisfying snack. They are known for being rich in vitamin E and a good source of calcium. They're also a good source of folate, magnesium, and fiber. A 2012 study found they have 20 percent fewer calories than previously calculated. They last up to a year in the refrigerator.

Hazelnuts—Also known as filberts, a serving is 21 nuts. The hazelnut grows in temperate climates and is the official state nut of Oregon, which grows 95 percent of the US commercial crop. They're rich in vitamin E, copper, and manganese, and a good source of magnesium and fiber. They can be stored up to three months out of the refrigerator, up to six months in the refrigerator, and up to a year frozen. Hazelnuts pair with savory, citrus, and sweet flavors.

Pine nuts—Also known as Indian nut, piñon, pinoli, and pignolia, pine nuts are the soft nuts found inside of pine cones. They are widely used in Mediterranean dishes and commonly used in the United States as a garnish or blended into pestos. Pine nuts are a good source of vitamin E and number 167 nuts per ounce.

Pistachios—California is one of the world's top pistachio producers and grows 98 percent of the US crop. A 2011 USDA study found that pistachios, known as the skinny nut for being one of the lowest fat, lowest calorie nuts, had 5 percent fewer calories than previously calculated. Pistachios are commonly consumed in-shell, and the simple act of shelling them leaves a visual cue for easy portion control. Their creamy shells naturally open when ripe, resembling a smile and earning them the nickname "smiling nut" in Iran and "happy nut" in China. Pistachios are the only green nut, owing to their carotenoids lutein and zeaxanthin. They're a good source of protein, fiber, magnesium, manganese, copper, thiamin, and phosphorus. There are 49 nuts in a serving.

Walnuts—The only nut with a significant amount of omega-3 fats, walnuts are rich in manganese and copper, and a good source of magnesium. The fertile land in California's Central Valley grows 99 percent of the US supply and three quarters of global trade. They can be stored in the refrigerator for up to three months and up to a year in the freezer. There are 14 halves per serving.

Other Nuts

Brazil nuts—There are six nuts per serving, as Brazils are large. As one might imagine from their name, these nuts grow in the Amazon. About 15 to 25 nuts grow inside a shell about the size of a coconut. They last out of the refrigerator in a cool, dry place for up to a month, or frozen for up to a year. Brazils are known for providing a full day's worth of selenium, an antioxidant. They're also rich in magnesium, copper, and phosphorus, and a good source of manganese, vitamin E, and thiamin.

Cashews—A single cashew nut dangles from an apple-shaped fruit before it is harvested. Soft with a delicate flavor, cashews are native to South America. Today, most are grown in India, Brazil, Vietnam, and Mozambique. They can be used to create creamy nut butters and vegan cheese. Cashews are rich in copper and a good source of magnesium, manganese, vitamin K, phosphorus, and zinc. They last in the refrigerator for up to six months, and up to a year frozen. There are 18 nuts per serving.

Macadamia nuts—There are 10 to 12 nuts per serving of these smooth, buttery nuts that grow natively in Australia and Hawaii. They're an excellent source of manganese and a good source of thiamin. They should be refrigerated and can last up to two months there, or in unopened, airtight containers for up to a year in the freezer.

Pecans—With 19 halves per serving, pecans are native to what is now the United States South. They are commonly used in sweets, but a healthier way to enjoy them is as a simple snack, a fish crust, or in a green salad. Pecans are rich in manganese, and a good source of copper, thiamin, and fiber. They last for up to six months refrigerated, and up to a year frozen.

Peanuts—Not technically a nut (they're a legume), they have many of the same properties and health benefits as tree nuts. They're an excellent source of manganese and a good source of folate, magnesium, phosphorus, vitamin E, and niacin. There are 28 kernels per serving.

Beans

The MIND diet recommends eating beans, a kind of legume, four times a week or more. Beans are rich in plant protein, fiber,

B vitamins, iron, potassium, and additional essential minerals. In addition to being nutrient-dense, they are low in total and saturated fat.

Diets higher in beans have been shown to slow cognitive decline. A study of more than 2,000 Swedish older adults aged 60 years and up showed that healthy diets that include beans provide neuroprotection. The same trend was found in a study of Taiwanese adults aged 65 years and up.

In addition to their contributions to brain health, beans belong in a healthy diet for their broad nutrition and health benefits. Beans have been positively associated with longevity in a cross-cultural study looking at food intake of adults aged 70 years and up from multiple cultures. This study found that for every 20 grams of beans eaten, the risk of mortality went down by 7 percent. Therefore, a half-cup serving of beans (85 grams) could reduce the risk of all-cause mortality by 30 percent.

Beans are also low-glycemic, slow-digesting carbohydrate foods, making them ideal for even blood sugar levels, and diabetes prevention and management. Their fiber and potassium are heart-healthy, and beans have been proven to improve cholesterol levels in people with heart disease. Last but not least, high-fiber foods—and beans definitely qualify—are identified as probable protectors against colon and rectal cancer by the World Cancer Research Fund International and the American Institute for Cancer Research.

Beans are in a family of foods that includes healthy choices such as lentils, peas, and peanuts. The top five beans eaten in the United States are pinto beans, which account for about half of all beans grown and eaten domestically, navy beans, black beans, garbanzo beans, and great northern beans. Generally speaking, beans are an excellent source of folate and provide manganese, magnesium, iron, plant protein, fiber, potassium, and other important nutrients.

Both plant protein and plant iron are more efficiently absorbed when eaten together with animal protein such as Pacific cod,

Alaskan salmon, or skinless chicken. Vitamin C from berries or vegetables also improves nutrient absorption. Combining these foods pulls even more nutrition out of beans.

All Forms Matter

Beans are available in fresh, dried, frozen, and canned forms. Cooked beans are available in BPA-free cans, as well as aseptic cartons, which are always BPA-free. For these kinds of packaged beans, drain and rinse them to remove about 40 percent of the sodium. For dried beans, the process requires some time, but is otherwise very simple: sort, rinse, soak, and cook (alternatively, skip the soak and cook low and slow for a longer period of time).

Dried beans are more affordable and closer to their natural state. They love moisture, low temperatures, and can stand up to long cooking times, making them ideal for slow-cooker dishes. Most dried beans need at least an hour to fully cook, though cranberry beans and great northern beans only need 45 to 60 minutes. Pink beans need about an hour. Black beans and small red beans need an hour to an hour and a half. The longest cooking beans need anywhere from an hour and a half to two hours, including dark red and light red kidney beans, navy beans, and pinto beans.

Get to Know Beans

Black beans—These get their deep dark color from anthocyanins, the same antioxidants that make blueberries blue. They are an excellent source of fiber, folate, iron, and magnesium. Black beans are commonly used in Caribbean, Central American, and South American recipes, and work well in salads, veggie burgers, and pureed into dips and soups. Cooking time: 60 to 90 minutes.

Cranberry beans—They are medium in size, oval in shape, and tan in color, streaked with cranberry red lines that disappear with cooking. They have a creamy texture and chestnut-like flavor, and are a favorite in northern Italy and Spain. They're also known as Roman beans. Cooking time: 45 to 60 minutes.

Green soybeans (edamame)—Rarely sold fresh, edamame is more commonly available frozen. If you find fresh edamame pods, keep them dry, in a perforated plastic bag, refrigerated, for up to four to five days. Edamame contains all nine essential amino acids, making it an excellent vegetarian protein source. It's also a good source of vitamin A, calcium, and iron.

Fava beans—Most often enjoyed fresh versus dried, fava beans should be in pods that are firm without too many markings. Pods should be heavy. They'll stay fresh for five to seven days in the refrigerator. They're an excellent source of fiber and folate, and can be enjoyed in hummus, soups, salads, or lightly sautéed with mushrooms for a delightful spring side dish.

Great northern beans—Medium in size and oval in shape with a delicate and thin white skin, they have a mild, light flavor, making them a good choice for someone new to beans. Great northern beans are often used in French and Mediterranean cuisine. They are smaller than cannellinis and are versatile: they can be used in salads, soups, stews, and purees. Cooking time: 45 to 60 minutes.

Red kidney beans—Kidney beans are relatively large, and as the name suggests, kidney-shaped. The red variety have a deep red, glossy skin and a firm texture that withstands long cooking times, making them a smart choice for slow-cooking dishes such as soups and chilis. Cooking time: 90 to 120 minutes.

Light red kidney beans—These are just like dark red kidney beans, except the skin is a glossy light red to pink hue. The light red variety are popular in Caribbean, Portuguese, and Spanish dishes. Both dark red and light red kidney beans can be used in Louisiana red beans and rice. Cooking time: 90 to 120 minutes.

Lima beans—Popular in Aztec and Inca cultures, lima beans are often in dried or canned forms. They are high in fiber and folate, and a good source of potassium and plant protein.

Navy beans—Navy beans are so called because they were a US Navy diet staple. They are small, white, oval-shaped beans with a mild and delicate flavor. Used in Boston baked beans, navy beans also work well in chilis, soups, and stews. They are rich in folate and fiber. Cooking time: 90 to 120 minutes.

Pink beans—This small, pink, oval-shaped bean is healthfully prepared in a popular Caribbean dish made with sofrito (a mixture of tomato, bell pepper, onions, and garlic), with no added fat. Cooking time: 60 minutes.

Pinto beans—These are medium, oval-shaped beans with mottled beige and brown skin similar to cranberry beans; and like cranberry beans, the streaks on dried pinto beans disappear during cooking. Pinto beans are very common and popular in the Americas and are used in Mexican refried beans, but a lighter way to enjoy them is in a side dish with diced red bell peppers, extra-virgin olive oil, lemon juice, red onion, and fresh pepper. Cooking time: 90 to 120 minutes.

Small red beans—As their name implies, they are small and red. They're oval in shape, softer and with a more delicate flavor than red kidney beans. They're often eaten with rice in Caribbean dishes. Cooking time: 60 to 90 minutes.

Berries

Berries are specifically included in the MIND diet, even though fruit in general is not. Berries have shown promise for both short- and long-term cognitive benefits.

Short-term experimental studies have shown that berries improve cognition, perhaps because berries are high in flavonoids, especially the kind called anthocyanidins, which have antioxidant and anti-inflammatory functions. Multiple animal studies have found that adding blueberries or strawberries to their diets reduced age-related declines in neural signaling and cognitive skills. In fact, in older rats, the neuronal and cognitive aging was reversed. In a study of older men with early cognitive impairments, adding blueberries or grape juice to their diets helped improve memory abilities.

A large, long-term study also points to the brain benefits of berries. Based on diet data that was collected over 21 years (1980–2001) from more than 16,000 women, a study in a subset of the Nurses' Health Study (NHS) found that total flavonoids, including anthocyanidins, can slow down the cognitive aging process by an average of up to two and a half years, and that berries were especially potent. Blueberries and strawberries were the most common sources of anthocyanidins in the diets of NHS participants.

People who ate blueberries once a week or more had better cognitive function, making them up to three and a half years younger than people who had a half cup or less per month. For strawberries, those who ate two or more servings per week were cognitively functioning up to three years younger than those who had less than a half cup per week.

For anthocyanidins, here are the top food sources:

- Blueberries

- Strawberries

- Apples

- Red wine

For total flavonoids, the top sources are:

- Tea (contributed one-half of all flavonoids in the study diet)

- Apples

- Oranges

- Onions

Note: This study didn't find any statistically significant connection to cognitive aging for any of the flavonoid foods individually, but it may be that total flavonoids are more important than any one source.

Pomegranate juice may also be a potent berry for brain health, with studies showing benefits in as little as four weeks. A UCLA study in older adults with mild age-related memory complaints, who were on average in their early 60s, tested a daily regimen of 8 ounces of pomegranate juice or a placebo for four weeks. The pomegranate juice group significantly improved verbal memory and had increased functional brain activity during the verbal and visual memory tasks. Pomegranate juice has more antioxidant potency than red wine and several juices (Concord grape juice, blueberry juice, cranberry juice, açai juice, apple juice, and orange juice), and drinking it increases levels of antioxidants circulating in the body.

Anthocyanidins in berries are capable of crossing the blood-brain barrier and finding their way to local brain regions used in learning and memory such as the hippocampus. More generally, many flavonoids can help reduce inflammation in the brain and spinal cord. Flavonoid-rich foods can also activate certain receptors and pathways that are believed to enhance memory and cognition.

The MIND diet recommends eating berries twice a week. Blueberries and strawberries are widely available and popular. There are many additional berries to try, especially in the summer when a wide variety are in season, at peak quality, and usually most affordable. At times when fresh isn't available or convenient, frozen, canned, dried, and 100 percent juice forms are options.

Most berries are highly perishable and should be stored in the refrigerator without anything heavy on top, which can lead to bruising and spoilage. Wash just before using.

Fall Berries

Barbados cherries—Native to the West Indies as well as Central and South America, these cherries grow well in tropical and subtropical areas, including Florida. They're an excellent source of vitamins A and C. Choose firm, red cherries with the stems still attached. They'll last in the refrigerator for up to five days, or can be frozen for six months.

Black crowberries—These small, black cold-loving berries grow in Alaska, Canada, Newfoundland, and Greenland, and are popular in northern Europe. They are packed with antioxidants, manganese, and vitamin C. Choosing crowberries is similar to choosing good blueberries. Look for firm, plump, dry berries that are dusty blue to black. They'll last up to two weeks in the refrigerator.

Cape gooseberries—They get their name from a light tan to brown papery "cape" that surrounds them and makes them look a little like tomatillos (see page 52). They are green when young, but ripen to yellow. They are tart and have a similar texture to cherries. They're an excellent source of vitamins A and C, potassium, copper, and fiber. Choose brightly colored gooseberries with dry capes, though the capes are sometimes removed before shipping. They can be stored in the refrigerator for up to a week.

Cranberries—A holiday favorite, cranberries are native to North America and are called cranberries because the flowers look like cranes. Cranberries are a good source of vitamin C and fiber and are quite hardy; they can be refrigerated for up to two months. Look for firm cranberries that aren't shriveled or browning.

Huckleberries—This Midwest favorite can be easily interchanged with blueberries, and even resembles blueberries. The huckleberry is wild and native to North America, and also goes by the names bilberry, wineberry, and dyeberry. Choose smooth berries without mold. Huckleberries are an excellent source of vitamin C and antioxidants, and are best stored frozen after washing and drying.

Pomegranate—see page 73.

Winter Berries

Pomegranates—An antioxidant powerhouse, each pomegranate contains hundreds of seeds, called arils, surrounded by red flesh, both of which are edible. Pomegranates are an excellent source of fiber, vitamins C and K, potassium, folate, and copper. Choose pomegranates that are plump, round, and heavy for their size. They can be stored in a cool, dry area for a month, or in the refrigerator for up to two months.

Red currants—Due to their tartness, red currants are commonly used in jams and pie fillings, though healthier ways to include them in the diet are in smoothies or in no-sugar-added sauces for chicken. They're an excellent source of vitamin C and antioxidants, and can be stored unwashed in the refrigerator for up to a week. Choose brightly colored berries without mold or soft spots.

Spring Berries

Barbados cherries—see page 72.

Lychee—Sometimes spelled litchi, this member of the soapberry family has roots in China that go back more than 2,000 years. They resemble large raspberries, but their skin is rough and inedible. The flesh inside is white with a single large seed. Choose fruit that is heavy for its size, and know that brown patches mean that the fruit inside will be sweeter. They can be refrigerated inside a plastic bag for up to 10 days. Lychee are an excellent source of vitamin C.

Strawberries—These popular berries are covered in about 200 tiny seeds per berry, and are rich in vitamin C and folate. They should be shiny, firm, and bright red with fresh green caps. Look out for shriveled or mushy berries. They can be stored in the refrigerator unwashed for one to three days.

Summer Berries

Barbados cherries—see page 72.

Black crowberries—see page 72.

Black currants—These berries look like small, round, dark grapes, though they are not nearly as sweet. Because of their tartness, they are usually used in jellies and jams, and could also be used in smoothies and sauces. They are an excellent source of vitamin C, fiber, potassium, and manganese. Look for dry, firm, round currants, and stay vigilant for signs of moldy or crushed berries. Sort through them at home, and store the good berries in the refrigerator, unwashed, for up to a week. They can also be stored frozen for up to a year.

Blackberries—Sometimes mistaken for black raspberries, the difference is that they have a solid center (raspberries are hollow). They're an excellent source of vitamin C and fiber, and can be stored, unwashed, for three to six days.

Blueberries—A good source of vitamin C and fiber, blueberries are highly researched due to their high antioxidant activity. Look for firm, plump, dry blueberries with a dusty blue color. They can be stored in the refrigerator for up to two weeks.

Boysenberries—A hybrid of raspberries and blackberries, boysenberries are reddish-purple. They're an excellent source of fiber, folate, manganese, and vitamin K. Look for shiny, plump, firm berries, and avoid any berries that look bruised or wet. Sort through them at home to remove any moldy berries, then refrigerate, unwashed, for up to a week.

Cherries—A summertime favorite, cherries are a good source of vitamin C and potassium. Look for firm, red cherries with good color and stems still attached. They'll last in the refrigerator for up to 10 days.

Sour cherries—More tart than the common cherry, sour cherries are an excellent source of vitamins A, C, and fiber, and can be stored, unwashed, for two to three days in the refrigerator. They can also be rinsed, deseeded, and frozen for later use. Look for clean, bright, shiny, plump berries without blemishes. They can be enjoyed fresh, but for those that don't prefer the tart flavor on its own, it can be balanced by adding to whole grain dishes.

Elderberries—These small, dark berries are an excellent source of fiber, vitamins A, C, and B6, and they provide vitamin E, copper, and iron, too. Look for firm berries with rich, dark color. Sort out any mushy berries at home and store the good, unwashed berries in the refrigerator for up to a week.

Loganberries—Named after a judge named Logan in Santa Cruz who grew them in his backyard in the late 19th century, loganberries should be shiny, plump, firm, and red. They can be stored in the refrigerator for up to a week, unwashed. Loganberries are rich in vitamin C, fiber, and manganese. They also provide vitamin K and folate.

Longans—Similar to lychee but smaller and with a smoother skin that is tan instead of red, longan also belongs to the soapberry family. They're an excellent source of vitamin C and can be stored in plastic bags in the refrigerator for up to a week. Look for longans with an intense tan color, which indicates they are ripe. They should be firm and free of bruising or blemishes.

Lychee—see page 73.

Mulberries—They resemble and can easily be substituted for blackberries. They are an excellent source of vitamin C and manganese, and also provide vitamin K and iron. Look for mulberries that are shiny, plump, and firm. Avoid any berries that are bruised or wet. They can be stored, unwashed, in the refrigerator for up to a week.

Strawberries—see page 73.

Raspberries—While commonly red, raspberries can be black, purple, and even golden in color. They're rich in vitamin C and fiber, and can be stored unwashed in the refrigerator for a day or two. Look for dry, plump, and firm berries; avoid wet or moldy ones.

Poultry

The MIND diet recommends eating poultry twice a week, specifically noting that it should not be fried. In addition to providing a healthy protein to the diet, lean poultry is a source of vitamin B12, an essential nutrient that has received a great amount of attention in scientific literature for its role in brain health.

Poultry provides high-quality protein that includes all of the essential amino acids, as well as iron and zinc, in forms that the body can readily absorb them (i.e., improves their bioavailability). Pairing poultry with plant foods that contain iron and zinc also helps make those nutrients more bioavailable.

While it is a healthy alternative to red meat, it is not an everyday food in the MIND diet. This is similar to its position in the plant-based Mediterranean and DASH diet patterns. The American Heart Association recommends poultry without the skin, baked or grilled, twice a week.

The most common poultry you'll find at the grocery store are chicken and turkey. Light meat (breast meat) is generally leaner than dark meat (thighs), and many cuts are available already skinless.

However, skin-on, bone-in, or whole birds are often more affordable, and just require a little extra prep time to remove skin and trim visible fat before eating. For ground chicken and turkey, choose at least 90 to 95 percent lean options.

For the time-pressed, most grocers offer whole rotisserie chicken that is hot, fully cooked, and ready to go. Some offer roasted turkey as well. A few cautions though: Seek out no-salt-added items, and avoid the options with words like "savory" or "juicy," which can be code for "pumped with added salt." At home, remove the skin and visible fat.

Another option some grocers offer is plain (versatile) grilled chicken in the refrigerated case that can be tossed into salads, stir-fry dishes, soups, and stews. Keep in mind that the trade-off for the convenience of letting someone else do the cooking for you is less control over food safety practices, so only buy from food providers you trust to minimize risk.

At home, refrigerate raw poultry in the coldest area of the refrigerator, which is normally on the bottom shelf, in the back, farthest from the door. It can be stored here for up to two days, or frozen for up to two months. Cooked poultry can be refrigerated for up to three days, or frozen for up to one month.

Fish

The MIND diet includes at least one fish meal a week that is not fried, which is simpler than the several fish meals per week required by the Mediterranean diet. The MIND diet recommends just one serving per week because the research did not show additional brain health benefits with higher levels of intake. Eating fish and omega-3 fats has been associated with lower risk of Alzheimer's disease and stroke. Fish is a direct source of omega-3s, including docosapentaenoic acid (DHA), which is especially important for cognitive development and a normally functioning brain.

Small studies have shown a modest cognitive benefit with one fish meal a week. Large-scale population studies in older populations in the United States (Chicago Health and Aging Project, or CHAP), the Netherlands (Rotterdam Study), and France (PAQUID study) have also shown that fish intake lowers the risk of Alzheimer's disease.

A large study of older Chicago residents explored the relationship between fish, omega-3s, and cognitive decline. They studied 3,718 adults aged 65 years and older who were part of CHAP over a period of six years. After six years, people eating fish once or twice a week slowed down their cognitive aging by 10 to 13 percent per year, or the equivalent to being three to four years younger.

Even though one fish meal per week is enough to lower the risk of dementia, there may be other reasons to enjoy fish more often for heart health and as a lean protein choice. A research review of nine population studies found that eating fish more often reduced the risk of stroke in a dose-response manner (that is, more fish, more benefits). The *Dietary Guidelines for Americans 2015–2020* recommends two fish meals per week, or about 8 ounces for the week.

SHOULD YOU BE WORRIED ABOUT MERCURY IN FISH?

Seafood is one of the healthiest foods around, but fish can also be a source of mercury, a known neurotoxin. Mercury can build up in a pregnant woman's body to levels that can put the developing child at risk for poor cognitive performance in attention, fine motor tests, language, visual-spatial skills, and verbal memory.

Mercury also builds up in fish over a time, from both natural and industrial sources in the environment. Thus, longer-living, larger fish like tuna, tilefish, swordfish, shark, and king mackerel will be higher in mercury than, say, scallops, salmon, shrimp, anchovies, or freshwater trout, which are smaller and shorter living.

Pregnant women and young children are cautioned by the FDA to avoid certain fish because of their mercury content and should seek out low-mercury options. However, for middle-aged and older men and women, health experts agree that the benefits far outweigh the risks.

Until recently, very little was known about how eating seafood affected the brain's level of mercury and disease markers for dementia. A 2016 study published in the *Journal of the American Medical Association* sought to lay this question to rest. Led by MIND diet researcher Dr. Martha Clare Morris, the study asked two questions: 1) Did eating seafood mean higher levels of mercury in the brain? and 2) Did either eating seafood or having certain brain mercury levels lead to any brain diseases?

The study population was a cross section of people from the Memory and Aging Project (MAP) in Chicago, who passed away between 2004 and 2013. Diet information was collected regularly as part of the MAP study, and out of 554 deceased participants, about half (48.4 percent) had brain autopsies. Not surprisingly, the researchers found that eating more seafood did indeed lead to higher levels of mercury in the brain. Surprisingly, when it came to Alzheimer's disease, eating more than one seafood meal per week was associated with healthier brains even with higher levels of mercury in the brain. The neuritic plaques and tangles were more sparse in the fish eaters than those who didn't eat fish, who tended to have more severe and widespread tangles and a higher concentration of brain plaques.

Study participants ate an average of one to three fish meals per week, and according to the National Marine Fisheries Service, the top 10 most commonly consumed fish in the United States already have low-to-moderate levels of mercury (shrimp, salmon, canned tuna, tilapia, pollock, pangasius, cod, catfish, crab, and clams). Therefore, it's hard to say whether these results would hold true if the study participants had eaten higher-mercury fish, more frequent fish meals, or both.

The take-home message is that moderate fish intake is a healthy choice for cognitive health. It is already well-established as a nutritious protein for heart health, diabetes, general health, and longevity. This study adds to the positive news by linking moderate fish intake with lower signs of Alzheimer's disease, even with higher brain levels of mercury that go up as fish intake goes up.

Is Fried Fish OK?

It's common knowledge that frying is not the healthiest way to prepare a meal, but sometimes the benefits of eating a healthy food outweigh the risks (case in point, see Should You Be Worried about Mercury in Fish?). However, in the case of frying, that does not seem to be the case. Frying reduces omega-3 fat levels and increases saturated fat intake. In a large study, the Cardiovascular Health Study (CHS), eating fish only reduced the risk of Alzheimer's disease if it was fatty fish, and there was no such benefit seen with fried fish. In another large study, the Women's Health Initiative Observational Study, women who ate five (or more) servings of fish per week cut their risk of heart failure by 30 percent, but only if it was baked or broiled fish. In fact, in the same study, women who ate fried fish one (or more) times per week increased their risk of heart failure by 50 percent.

Finding Fresh Fish

Choosing fresh fish is simple with a few key tips. For whole fish, look for red gills (not brown), shiny metallic skin, and clear, bright eyes, both of which fade or dull when a fish has passed its peak. Gently press into the flesh of the fish and see how quickly the indentation disappears. Fresh fish has firm and resilient flesh without any gaps between layers. If there is liquid on the fish, it should run clear and not milky, which is an early sign of rotting. Lastly, fish should smell like clean ocean water (saltwater fish) or a clean pond (freshwater fish), but never pungent or "fishy."

Starter Seafood

If seafood isn't yet a regular part of your diet or you aren't sure it's your favorite, try starting with a mild, flaky white fish such as Pacific cod or halibut. These fish are buttery and delicate, and pick up the flavors they're cooked with, making them perfect for a gentle introduction to the wide world of seafood. Another great option is to mash anchovies and incorporate them into pasta sauces, which adds savory flavor without adding a fishy taste.

Frozen and canned fish are conveniently available year-round when fresh fish isn't practical.

What a recipe calls for and what's available at your local store may not always match up. Check out the chart below to see what types of fish are interchangeable.

EASY FISH SWAPS	
DESCRIPTION	**TYPES OF FISH**
White, lean, flaky	Atlantic croaker, black sea bass, branzino (aka European sea bass), flounder, rainbow smelt, red snapper, tilapia, rainbow trout, weakfish (sea trout), whiting
White, lean, firm	Alaska pollock, catfish, grouper, haddock, Pacific cod, Pacific halibut, Pacific rockfish, Pacific sand dab and sole, striped bass (wild and hybrid), swordfish
White, firm, oily	Atlantic shad, Albacore tuna, California white sea bass, Chilean sea bass, cobia, lake trout, lake whitefish, Pacific escolar, Pacific sablefish, white sturgeon
Medium and oily	Amberjack, Arctic char, Hawaiian kampachi, mahimahi, paddlefish, pompano, salmon (coho or sockeye), wahoo
Dark and oily	Anchovies, blue fin tuna, grey mullet, herring (Atlantic, Boston, or king), salmon (farmed or king/Chinook), sardines, skipjack, tuna

Sustainable Seafood

There are a number of ways to identify sustainably harvested (for farmed) and caught (for wild) fish. There is some confusion over wild versus farmed fish and what is more environmentally friendly. Unfortunately, there is no simple rule about what's better. There are damaging practices in both farmed and wild caught seafood. Sometimes the issue is that the population of the fish species is low, other times it may be that the way its caught catches and kills other species, or the way its farmed breeds disease and pollutes the water. These are just a few of the concerns.

It's a lot to keep track of, but that's exactly what credible scientific organizations such as the Safina Center in New York and Monterey Bay Aquarium in California do. They provide good general recommendations, and for additional assurances, there are trustworthy certifications given by the Marine Stewardship Council (for wild fish) and Aquaculture Stewardship Council (for farmed fish). This is an evolving issue, and as fish populations grow stronger or fish are caught or grown in more responsible ways, some fish may move from the "do not eat" to the "go ahead and enjoy" category.

Olive Oil

Similar to the Mediterranean diet, the MIND diet uses olive oil as its main fat. Olive oil boasts approximately 230 antioxidants and polyphenols. While the whole is more than its parts, it's possible that one such part, oleocanthal, has an especially protective role in brain health. Oleocanthal is one of hundreds of natural phenolic compounds in extra-virgin olive oil with antioxidant and anti-inflammatory properties. In an animal study published in *ACS Chemical Neuroscience*, oleocanthal helped shuttle abnormal proteins (beta-amyloid) out of the brain. The accumulation of beta-amyloid proteins form plaques that eventually disrupt nerve cell function, leading to the death of the affected brain cells, which is believed to be culprit in Alzheimer's disease. Oleocanthal boosted production of proteins and enzymes that are essential to removing beta-amyloid from the brain. In a sub-study of the larger PREDIMED trial, people eating diets supplemented with olive oil were associated with better immediate and delayed forms of verbal memory.

The MIND diet has no restriction on total fat and recommends olive oil as the main source of fat, especially in place of solid fats like butter, stick margarine, lard, and coconut oil. In the Mediterranean diet, it's not uncommon to consume 2 to 3 tablespoons per day, and the PREDIMED study recommends about 4 tablespoons of olive oil per day.

Extra-virgin olive oil, which is simply pressed olives, is special because it provides vitamins E and K, plus protective polyphenols. The most important things to know are that extra-virgin olive oil isn't for cooking, and all olive oil should come in dark or opaque containers to preserve the quality of the oil, as it breaks down with heat and light.

Extra-virgin olive oil is a finishing oil and should be enjoyed in salad dressings and on top of soups, toasts, and other dishes. It's not meant to be heated to high temperatures, which destroys the complex flavor that comes from the polyphenols and other phytonutrients; these, in turn, are what drive a premium price. Use regular olive oil for cooking, but even then, use it for low-heat cooking due to its relatively low smoke point (the temperature at which the oil begins to smoke and degrade into damaging free radicals). Going above the smoke-point causes damage to the oil that in turn can make it unhealthy to consume. For high-heat cooking, try a grapeseed oil, or a blend of olive oil with another vegetable oil.

Heat and light, as well as water and air, are enemies to all cooking oils. Olive oil, with its many phytonutrients, is no different. Look for containers that are dark glass, tin, or even clear glass, but then mostly covered with a label or box to protect the oil and its polyphenols from going bad too quickly. Store it in a cool, dark place away from the stove. It can be refrigerated, but it's not recommended, especially for higher-quality olive oils. Buy the right size of olive oil that will be used in a couple of months. This may mean buying smaller containers of olive oil to ensure it's being used at its best.

Find Good-Quality Olive Oil

Look for a harvest date. Good producers will include a date on the olive oil bottle indicating when the olives were harvested. Try to pick out an oil that's within a year of its harvest. The closer to the harvest date the better. Northern Hemisphere olives (e.g., from California, Spain, Italy, and Greece) are usually harvested in November to December, and Southern Hemisphere olives (e.g., from Argentina, Australia, Chile, and Peru) are typically harvested in May to June. Depending on the time it takes to process and bottle the oil, choosing olive oils closer to their harvest date may mean looking for California olive oil earlier in the year, and Australian olive oil in the second half of the year. The harvest date is not a "best by" date, which is often two years from the time the bottle was filled, not when the olives were harvested or processed.

Taste for freshness. Olive oil should taste vegetal or "green," slightly bitter, and have a peppery kick you can feel at the back of your throat when swallowing (this is a sign of healthy polyphenols in the oil, and a cough is not an uncommon first reaction). A quality olive oil can have fruity notes that range from grassy to apple to green banana and artichoke. It should not taste musty, metallic, or buttery, nor should it taste or smell like wine or vinegar.

Look for quality assurances. Recently, olive oil fraud has become an issue as manufacturers mix olive oil with colorings, flavors, and less expensive oils. In response to the questions about olive oil authenticity, some industry standards have emerged from the California Olive Oil Council (COOC) and the Australian Olive Oil Association (AOOA), which offer quality seals to identify olive oils that meet higher-quality standards than the minimal USDA ones.

A World of Flavors and Acidity

Olive oils are graded by acidity level, and the best ones are cold-pressed, which is a chemical-free process that simply involves pressure and results in a naturally low level of acidity. This is the way in which extra-virgin olive oil is made, resulting in a 1 percent acidity oil. It can be dark green to light champagne in color, with the darker-color oils offering the most intense olive flavors.

Italian olive oil tends to be dark green and has an herbal and grassy scent and flavor. Greek olive oil also tends to be green and is marked by strong flavors and aromas. Spain is one of the world's largest olive oil producers, and their olive oil commonly appears golden yellow and tastes both fruity and nutty. In contrast, French olive oil tends to be pale and mild in flavor. California olive oil also tends to be light in color and flavor, but with a fruitier taste. Any of these can be of extra-virgin quality.

Virgin olive oil is also a first-press oil, but the level of acidity is slightly higher, in the 1 to 3 percent range. Oils simply labeled as "olive oil" could be a mix of refined olive oil and virgin or extra-virgin olive oil. It used to be called "pure" olive oil. Light olive oil is a refined olive oil that is light in flavor and color, not calories. Light olive oil has a higher smoke point than regular olive oil, so it's better for low- and medium-heat cooking.

Wine

The MIND diet includes a glass of wine a day, no more, no less. Wine is a polyphenol-rich food that has been associated with better cognitive function in a recent sub-study of the larger PREDIMED trial. In the sub-study of 447 older men and women ages 55 to 80 years, those who drank wine scored better on the mini–mental state exam, a 30-point set of questions that test a range of everyday mental skills, from being able to identify the correct year, spell a word backward, remember a series of words mentioned earlier, repeat phrases, and more.

While observational studies suggest moderate alcohol intake reduces the risk of Alzheimer's disease, they also point to high intakes increasing the risk. A recent review of research that's current up to September 2011 on alcohol, dementia, and pre-dementia suggests that the protective effects of moderate alcohol intake, such as the one glass of wine a day in the MIND diet, are more promising in people without the common genetic marker for Alzheimer's disease, APOE-e4. It's also more promising for wine compared to other types of alcohol. This same paper concludes that there are no signs light drinking would be harmful to cognition and dementia.

Red wine contains resveratrol and other polyphenols, which are antioxidants and anti-inflammatory. As potent antioxidants, they may help, in conjunction with a diet rich in polyphenols, to reduce and protect against the formation of the beta-amyloid plaques that come with Alzheimer's disease.

What if you don't prefer wine or alcohol in general? Interestingly, a study of alcohol-free wine found that it was an excellent source of antioxidants, and that it was effective in increasing antioxidant activity. The PREDIMED study only included one daily glass of wine for those who already drank wine regularly; even then, it was optional.

A serving size is 5 ounces (be mindful, as today's glassware often holds multiple servings). When it comes to the best way to incorporate wine with food, the first rule to live by is to drink according to your preferences, and let your own palate and budget be your guide. Other than that, there are a few guiding principles of how to pair food and wine, but these are just suggestions. Below are some recommendations for wines that generally pair well with the brain-healthy foods in the MIND diet.

Vegetables—Raw vegetables, such as those in a crudités platter, go well with white wines such as chardonnay, pinot blanc, and chenin blanc. Asparagus goes great with white wines such as sauvignon blanc and dry Riesling. Stir-fry vegetables with East Asian flavor (e.g., soy, rice vinegar, chili) is complemented by slightly sweet German Rieslings.

Nuts—The savory-rich flavors and mouthfeel of heart-healthy fats from nuts goes well with dry (brut) sparkling wines and champagne. Nuts can also stand up to the richness of a fortified wine such as port.

Beans—Pairing wine with beans is more about what kind of bean is used and how it is prepared. Generally, mild white beans will work with white wines, and headier and hardier beans that may be used in chilis will work better with reds. Summer recipes may work best with chardonnay or rose, and richer recipes may work better with reds.

Berries—It's true: strawberries and champagne are a match made in heaven. Generally, berries pair well with sparkling wines—from dry to semi-dry, as well as sweeter white wines like Riesling and muscat. To try something a little different, pair berries with a light red wine like zinfandel.

Poultry—Chicken is versatile, and so are the wines that pair with it, from white wines like chardonnay, vin gris, Riesling, and chenin blanc to lighter reds like merlot and pinot noir. Chicken dishes made with savory tomatoes and mushrooms may work best with a light red wine; chicken made with brighter flavors such as ginger, garlic, or lemon may work best with white wines. A picnic-worthy chicken salad would work nicely with slightly sweeter white wines such as Riesling or gewürztraminer. Turkey pairs nicely with red wines such as merlot and zinfandel, and with white wines such as chardonnay.

Fish—Tuna goes well with white wine, such as sauvignon blanc. The richness of salmon pairs well with pinot noir as well as some white wines, from pinot gris to sauvignon blanc. The fresh, clean flavors of sashimi generally pair well with dry sparkling wine, dry

Riesling, or a soft red like pinot noir or beaujolais. However, the wines that work best with specific types of sushi may vary.

Whole grains—Whole grain pasta salad goes well with white wines such as sauvignon blanc and dry Rieslings. If the pasta is prepared with tomato sauce, a light red wine may work better, such as a zinfandel.

Olive oil—Similar to nuts, the velvety mouthfeel of heart-healthy fats from olive oil goes well with dry (brut) sparkling wines and champagne.

By the glass—If, instead, you are starting with a bottle of wine and are looking for inspiration on what to make for dinner that may go well with it, here are a few guidelines.

White	*Champagne* for savory foods
	Sauvignon blanc for tart dressings and sauces (citrus, vinegar)
	Gruner veltliner with herbs
	Pinot grigio with light dishes
	Chardonnay with fatty fish or fish in a rich sauce
	Slightly sweet *Riesling* with sweet and spicy dishes such as Asian dishes (also applies to *gewürztraminers* and *vouvrays*)
	Moscato d'asti for fruit desserts
Rose/Reds	*Rose champagne* for hors d'oeuvres and dinner, it's versatile
	Pinot noir with earthy flavors like mushrooms and bitter vegetables
	Malbec and spicy dishes as its bold enough to withstand strong flavors
	Syrah for spicy dishes

Finally, remember that these are broad guidelines, and that your preferences may be very different. In addition, if dining out, a sommelier can share more specific recommendations for wine pairings and menu items.

CHAPTER 4
Brain-Harming Foods

The MIND diet's five types of brain-harming foods are red meat, butter and stick margarine, whole-fat cheese, pastries and sweets, and fried fast foods. Limiting these foods was part of the diet that led to better cognitive aging and reduced the risk of Alzheimer's disease in the MIND studies. The MIND researchers note that these are all foods that increase the intake of saturated and trans fats in proportion to unsaturated fats, which leads to blood-brain barrier problems and increases beta-amyloid plaque. In addition, two of the food groups—pastries and sweets and fried fast food—provide little nutrition, and most generally healthy diets recommend limiting them.

The MIND diet advice to avoid saturated fat agrees with the recent *Dietary Guidelines for Americans 2015–2020*, which recommends limiting saturated fat to less than 10 percent of total calories (22 grams or less in a 2000-calorie diet). The human body makes all the saturated fat it needs, which means there is zero biological need to have any saturated fat in the diet. According to the government report, there is strong and consistent evidence that replacing saturated fat with unsaturated fat—especially the polyunsaturated type—lowers LDL (bad) cholesterol and heart attacks. Similar evidence exists for the benefits of eating monounsaturated fats such as olive oil and nuts instead of saturated fat from foods like butter, margarine, beef, whole-fat cheese, sweets, and fried fast food.

Current research suggests saturated fat may be neutral when it comes to heart disease, usually when it replaces a refined carbohydrate. What we do know is that countless studies show that replacing saturated fat with polyunsaturated fat reduces heart disease risk. In addition, there are several studies in the area of cognitive decline and Alzheimer's disease suggesting an increased risk coming from too much saturated fat in the diet. Regardless of whether saturated fat is neutral instead of harmful, there are healthier fats to include in the diet. Unsaturated fats are found in nuts, fish, and olive oil.

Five Food Groups to Avoid

Red Meat

Red meat includes beef, lamb, duck, and pork. They may be in meat products such as hamburgers, beef tacos and burritos, hot dogs, sausages, meatballs, meatloaf, and deli meats.

The MIND diet recommends limiting red meat to fewer than four times per week. The World Health Organization classified processed meat as a group 1 carcinogen in October 2015 (the same category as tobacco and asbestos), noting that evidence suggests red meat probably is too. Being designated as a "group 1 carcinogen" is the strongest rating, and means there is convincing evidence that the substance causes cancer.

The damaging effects are seen over many meals, days, weeks, and years. A 2015 study of Taiwanese adults aged 65 years and up found that typical Western eating patterns high in meat increased the risk of cognitive decline over eight years compared to a healthy diet that included vegetables, beans, fish, fruit, and legumes. Over the eight-year period, a Western dietary pattern nearly tripled the risk of cognitive decline. A multi-decade study of more than 120,000 men and women, conducted by Harvard researcher Frank Hu and his team, estimated that swapping out a serving of red meat each day with healthier protein options such as fish, poultry, nuts, beans, low-fat dairy, and whole grains could lower the risk of death by 7 to 19 percent.

If you don't already enjoy red meat, there's no reason to start. But if you do choose to eat red meat occasionally, follow these basic rules to do it in the healthiest way possible:

- Choose the least processed meat possible. That means choosing fresh cuts of meat versus processed meat like bacon, beef jerky, bologna, canned meat, ham, hot dogs, mortadella, pastrami, pepperoni, salami, and sausages. Many deli meats fall into this category, though sliced lunch meat that is simply cooked and sliced isn't considered processed, such as roast beef, turkey, and chicken.

- Opt for grass-fed, organic meat. It tends to be leaner and has a different nutrient profile due to the grass-based diet, including more carotenoids, vitamin E, potassium, iron, and zinc than conventional meat.

- Look for fresh meat at the grocery store that is labeled as "lean" or "extra lean." Choose cuts that are "choice" or "select" over fattier cuts labeled as "prime."

- For ground meats, look for the lowest percentage of fat, such as "95 percent lean meat, 5 percent fat."

Beef—"Extra lean" cuts of beef are eye round roast/steak, sirloin tip side steak, top round roast/steak, bottom round roast/steak, and top sirloin steak.

Bison—Sirloin, rib eye, and top round cuts all have 2 grams of fat per serving.

Veal—leg, sirloin, and loin all have 3 grams or less fat per serving.

Pork—tenderloin has 2 grams fat per serving and sirloin cuts have about 4 grams of fat per serving.

Lamb—lamb shank, loin, and shoulder have 6 grams of fat or less per serving.

Butter and Stick Margarine

The MIND diet recommends limiting butter and stick margarine to less than a tablespoon per day. Generally, any fat that is solid at room temperature has too much saturated fat to be included in the MIND diet, including the butter and stick margarine already mentioned, but also palm oil, coconut oil, beef tallow, lard, and shortening.

The MIND diet encourages using olive oil as the main fat. However, if you love butter and stick margarine as a spread, there are vegetable oil spreads available with lower saturated fat and zero trans fat.

WHAT ABOUT COCONUT OIL?

Coconut oil has made headlines recently as a miracle food, despite its high saturated fat content. The theory behind why coconut oil may have benefits is based on its high percentage of medium-chain triglycerides, or MCTs. This type of fat is metabolized differently than the long-chain triglycerides (LCT) that make up the majority of liquid oils. The idea is that MCT goes directly from the intestine to the liver, so less is available to be stored as body fat, but studies using coconut oil haven't shown meaningful weight loss. It should be noted that when modest weight loss (around 4 pounds) has been seen, it is when man-made, formulated 100 percent MCT replaces another oil (coconut oil is about 40 percent LCT and 60 percent MCT).

There is also no good evidence that virgin coconut oil is healthier for the heart compared to conventional coconut oil. However, when coconut oil is referred to as "virgin," it generally means it's less processed compared to common coconut oil, which may be bleached, deodorized, or refined. Unlike olive oil, there is no industry standard for what virgin means when it comes to coconut oil.

Nutrition science is an evolving field, but what we do know today is that there isn't enough evidence to support that coconut oil is effective for the many ailments it claims to help, including Alzheimer's disease, heart disease, obesity, or diabetes. It is interesting that there are contradicting studies on how it affects LDL (good) and HDL (bad) cholesterol, but the data is inconclusive at this time.

Cheese

The MIND diet recommends limiting whole-fat cheese to less than one serving a week. The *Dietary Guidelines for Americans 2015–2020* and the American Heart Association recommend limiting it in a heart-healthy diet. The Dietary Guidelines recommend choosing fat-free or low-fat milk and yogurt instead of whole-fat cheese to reduce saturated fat and sodium intake while benefiting from vitamins A and D, and potassium in dairy foods.

Vegan cheeses offer a cholesterol-free option, though they may still be high in saturated fat. Take a look at the nutrition facts panel for more details and look for a saturated fat amount listed at below 10 percent of the Daily Value.

Pastries and Sweets

The MIND diet recommends limiting pastries and sweets to fewer than five times per week. The *Dietary Guidelines for Americans 2015–2020* discourages eating these foods not only because of their bad fats, but also because of their added sugar. These foods offer little to no positive nutrients. There is no need for these foods within a healthy diet, and they should only be included in very limited amounts.

Pastries and sweets include cookies, cakes, brownies, cupcakes, croissants, doughnuts, custards, ice cream, candy, and more. In addition to pastries and sweets, sugar-sweetened beverages such as soda, sports drinks, and juice that is not 100 percent juice should be limited.

Satisfy your sweet tooth naturally with whole fruit. They naturally contain sugars but in a reasonable ratio to their fiber, water, and total package of nutrition. In fact, berries such as blueberries and strawberries are sweet, nutritious, and an important component of the MIND diet.

Fried Fast Food

The MIND diet recommends limiting fried fast food to less than one serving per week. That means, at the most, having fried fast food once every two weeks, or about twice a month. The *Dietary Guidelines for Americans 2015–2020* recommends limiting fried foods because frying diminishes the healthfulness of any food. In fact, frying dilutes the nutrition in otherwise healthy foods such as poultry, fish, and vegetables, negating their brain health benefits.

If you find yourself at a fast food chain, you can still make smart choices. Look for the healthiest options on the menu. It may be a salad, with toppings and dressing on the side so you can choose whether and how much to consume. It may be a grilled chicken or grilled fish sandwich on whole wheat bread. Instead of French fries or chips, some chains offer healthier sides such as baby carrots. If you are served something with fried breading, you can remove it before eating.

Many of the larger chains offer nutrition information on site and online and must produce it on request so you can make informed choices.

CHAPTER 5

The Nutrients

Nutrients will never trump whole foods, but understanding how key nutrients function still helps improve the understanding of how foods work to improve health. It's an imperfect set of knowledge to begin with, and this chapter is not exhaustive. Instead, it is meant to provide an overview of some of the best-studied and most promising nutrients that are involved in cognitive aging, dementia, and cognitive development, from nutrients with antioxidant and anti-inflammatory action to those with a possible role in protecting against beta-amyloid deposits and cell death. This includes dietary fats, vitamin E, certain B vitamins (folate and B12), flavonoids, and carotenoids.

When thinking about individual nutrients distilled into supplements, it is important to understand the well-established nutrition principle that the intersection of nutrients and health fall on a U-shaped curve where getting too little leads to deficiency, and too much leads to toxicity. Good health is in between the extremes. Supplements can easily go overboard on nutrients, whereas food sources won't. That's why, with a few exceptions, taking a food-first approach is the ideal way for older adults to meet nutrient needs.

Good and Bad Fats

There is no max on total fat in the MIND diet, but the types and proportions of fats matter.

Good Fats

The PREDIMED trial tested a Mediterranean diet supplemented with healthy fats, either nuts or olive oil, and both were effective in producing higher cognitive scores compared to low-fat diets. Risk for Alzheimer's disease and cognitive decline goes down when unsaturated fats replace saturated and trans fats.

The MIND diet emphasizes the use of olive oil as the main dietary fat. It is rich in monounsaturated fat as well as many polyphenols. Other sources of healthy fats include nuts, seeds, avocado, and vegetable oil.

Bad Fats

Eating too much saturated and trans fats increases the risk of dementia. When it comes to unhealthy fats, research shows that diets high in saturated and trans fats lead to signs of dementia such as blood-brain barrier dysfunction, inflammation, and amyloid clusters. Several observational studies have also found that middle-age adults with high cholesterol are at an increased risk of developing dementia later in life.

In one animal study, there was significant blood-brain barrier damage and inflammation after three months on a diet high in saturated fat. The functional damage was 30 times worse than at the start. The diet used in the study was 20 percent saturated fat, which equates to a little more than 44 grams of saturated fat for a 2,000-calorie diet. In another animal study, amyloid concentrations went up as a result of four months on a diet that was 40 percent saturated fat (nearly 90 grams of saturated fat for a 2,000 calorie diet). In a cell study, trans fat was found to favor the formation of sticky amyloid proteins seen in Alzheimer's disease while also discouraging a variation of the protein that does not result in amyloids. Studies also suggest that high-fat diets, especially when high in saturated fat, affect cognitive performance. Learning and memory skills declined in a long-term animal study of mice eating a diet that was 40 percent fat (versus 4.5 percent in the standard food). Based on nearly two decades of research in this area, the scientists concluded that a long-term high-fat diet disrupts the way the body uses glucose: the hippocampus region of the brain adapts to use less of it.

The easiest way to avoid saturated and trans fat is to avoid the brain-harming foods identified in the MIND diet. Another way to easily identify a saturated fat is to see if it is solid at room temperature.

Good vs. Bad Fats

In the research that adjusted for types of fat, results were consistent: the more saturated and trans fats there were in the diet, the higher the rates of cognitive decline. In addition, most of these studies found that higher intakes of monounsaturated (MUFA) and polyunsaturated (PUFA) fats did the reverse and led to a slowdown of cognitive decline. These findings are supported by lab studies in which animals eating diets higher in omega-3s (especially DHA, which is abundant in brain tissue), including older mice, did better at learning new things and remembering.

Why do some studies show mixed results? Some randomized trials using DHA omega-3 supplements didn't show any benefits for cognitive health. These trials allowed participants to eat fish up to three times per week, so the difference between treatment and placebo groups would have been nullified given that just one fish meal per week is adequate for reducing risk of dementia. There are also mixed results from several population studies of dietary fat and cognitive decline, but only when the methodology did not control for type of fat.

Vitamin E

MIND diet foods that are naturally rich in vitamin E include olive oil, nuts, whole grains, and green, leafy vegetables. Vitamin E is important to brain health. As an antioxidant nutrient, it protects the brain from the oxidative stress and damage to neural tissue that comes with being a site of high metabolic activity. A deficiency in this essential nutrient leads to a variety of brain-related symptoms, including cognitive decline, loss of control over the body's movement, lack of reflexes, paralyzed eye muscles, and decreased sensitivity to vibration, all of which decrease the ability to fully function in society.

Naturally occurring vitamin E comes in eight forms, but for our purposes we'll focus on the two most commonly studied ones, referred to by their chemical names: alpha-tocopherol and gamma-tocopherol. Both of these forms are found in food, and have antioxidant and anti-inflammatory properties. However, the vitamin E appearing on nutrition labels refers to alpha-tocopherol. It's also the most common form found in dietary supplements. It is considered to be the most biologically active and is the only form with a recommended intake level for general health established by the Institute of Medicine, part of the National Academies of Sciences, Engineering, and Medicine.

Animal research has shown that vitamin E protects the brain against Alzheimer's disease. Epidemiological studies consistently show benefits of dietary (food-sourced) vitamin E for Alzheimer's prevention. However, several studies using a vitamin E supplement found no benefit, and even some harm for cognitive decline and Alzheimer's disease.

A 2015 research study published in *Alzheimer's & Dementia* is the only human study on vitamin E in the brain and Alzheimer's disease. It helps explain the confusion around the mixed results, ultimately concluding that the more gamma-tocopherol vitamin

E (found in foods such as pistachios) there was in the brain, the healthier it looked. Higher levels of gamma-tocopherol in the brain were associated with lower levels of amyloid and neurofibrillary tangles.

The confusion around vitamin E's brain-health benefits is due to several studies on vitamin E supplements (in the form of alpha-tocopherol), which show no benefits for cognitive decline or Alzheimer's disease. These null results were supported by observational epidemiological studies (the kind of studies that follow large groups of people over several years) that looked at vitamin E supplementation and cognitive decline. These results were disappointing, especially after many animal studies had shown that alpha-tocopherol supported brain health. The few studies showing brain-protective effects of alpha-tocopherol supplementation were for people who started with low levels of vitamin E in their diet. Levels of vitamin E would need to be below 6.1 milligrams per day (about 9 IU) in order for supplements to have a positive effect, according to an analysis of nutrient insufficiency in older adult populations.

The bottom line is that vitamin E from foods is preferable to vitamin E from supplements, which may do more harm than good, and at best, are still controversial. There is no controversy around vitamin E from foods, and both alpha-tocopherol and gamma-tocopherol from foods reduced the rate of cognitive decline and Alzheimer's disease. The key difference is that the amounts found in foods are at much more moderate levels and work together to keep the brain healthy. Furthermore, foods may contain more of the eight vitamin E forms, not just the two that have been well studied. These other forms are also known to have antioxidant and anti-inflammatory properties. These provide all the more reason to choose food first and to be cautious of reducing the benefits of whole foods to single nutrients. Natural sources of vitamin E include whole grains, nuts, and vegetable oils.

WHAT DOES VITAMIN E ON A LABEL MEAN?

Vitamin E on food or supplement labels only refers to alpha-tocopherols and may be listed in milligrams (mg), which is a measure of quantity. It will more likely be listed in international units (IU), which is a measure of biological activity.

For natural vitamin E, every milligram equals 1.49 international units. If natural vitamin E is shown in IU, simply multiply by 0.67 to get the amount in milligrams.

Synthetic vitamin E is less bioavailable, and a milligram equals 2.22 IU. To convert IU of synthetic vitamin E to milligrams, multiply by 0.45. The daily value for natural vitamin E is 30 IU, which is approximately 20 milligrams of natural alpha-tocopherols. People need about 50 percent more IU of synthetic vitamin E (e.g., through supplements or fortified foods) to get the same amount as the natural form.

What else does vitamin E do for health? Vitamin E is an essential nutrient that the body cannot produce on its own (which is why it must come from the diet). It is an antioxidant, which means it protects the body against damage caused by free radicals. It helps keep the immune system strong, helps form red blood cells, helps the body use vitamin K, and assists in widening the blood vessels to keep blood from clotting inside them. Vitamin E is a fat-soluble vitamin, which means that the body needs dietary fat to absorb it.

Healthy eating patterns should include at least 20 percent of calories from fat, without which it's hard to meet recommended intake levels of important fat-soluble nutrients. In any case, type of fat is more important than total fat, as long as a certain minimum is met (the 20 percent) and it's within calorie needs. The *Dietary Guidelines for Americans 2015–2020*, which de-emphasizes total fat limits and focuses more on the type of fat, recommends eating many foods that contain both healthy fats and vitamin E, such as vegetable oils, nuts, and seeds. Vitamin E is also commonly found in green, leafy vegetables. Specific examples of natural food sources include olive oil, almonds, pistachios, peanuts, sunflower seeds, beet greens, collard greens, spinach, and broccoli. The recommended daily value is 30 IU, with upper limits set at 1,500 IU per day for natural forms and 1,000 IU per day for synthetic forms. Eating vitamin E in foods is safe, but higher doses from supplements can increase the risk of bleeding in general, bleeding in the brain, and birth defects.

B Vitamins: Folate and B12

Folate (vitamin B9) and vitamin B12 (cobalamin) are both essential, water-soluble B vitamins that are often discussed together because they are involved in many of the same functions and are interrelated. Without enough of either, the body's red blood cell count goes down, reducing the ability to deliver oxygen to tissues. Vitamin B12 deficiency can result in cognitive impairment as well as fatigue, depression, anemia, and nerve damage that can cause tingling, numbness, burning, and loss of feeling in arms, hands, legs, and feet (also known as peripheral neuropathy). They are both involved in brain development early in life, as well as brain degeneration later in life.

These two vitamins are studied in relation to dementia because they help metabolize homocysteine, a substance that has been associated with an increased risk of developing Alzheimer's disease. Without enough folate and B12 in the diet, homocysteine accumulates in the body. B vitamin supplementation (folate, B12, and B6) was shown to be helpful in a study that targeted older adults with high homocysteine. Two years of treatment slowed down overall cognitive decline, including memory complaints.

However, the body of research on these two vitamins and dementia has been complicated by inconsistent findings. Ten population studies have looked at folate and B12 in relation to cognitive decline. Three showed protective effects for B12, and four had positive results for folate, but several had mixed results.

A 2012 paper by Dr. Martha Clare Morris, published in *Proceedings of the Nutrition Society*, describes methodology issues resulting in study designs that are not sensitive enough to show an effect. Some studies did not measure participants' starting levels for these nutrients, which is important because supplementation may only benefit people who have a need (that is, those with low B vitamin status). For example, among several large, long-term trials, one took starting folate levels into account, and when low-folate status was identified, there was a benefit from folic acid supplementation, resulting in a slower rate of cognitive decline. In a study that found no overall effect for B vitamin supplementation, there actually was a protective benefit when a later analysis of the data focused on participants who had low B vitamin levels at the start of the study.

Is It Possible to Get Too Much Folate?

Folic acid is the synthetic form of folate, and deficiency is now rare since the USDA mandated folic acid fortification of grains in 1998. They did so in response to the well-established role of folate in preventing fetal neural tube defects, and there's good evidence it helped dramatically reduce cases by 36 percent in its first 10 years (1996–2006). However, an unintended consequence is that older adults may be getting too much.

Folate, a water-soluble vitamin, isn't usually stored in the body; excesses are removed in the urine. However, some research shows that the liver doesn't easily metabolize folic acid (the form used in fortified foods and supplements) into the form of folate the body can use, resulting in high levels of unmetabolized folic acid circulating in the blood. A study among CHAP participants found that people with folic acid intakes above the recommended daily

400 micrograms experienced faster cognitive decline. Similar results were reported in a study of the large National Health and Nutrition Examination Survey (NHANES) data, in which low B12 and high folate led to impaired cognitive performance compared to people with normal levels of folate.

Is it possible to get too much vitamin B12 from supplements? Vitamin B12 from food isn't well-absorbed by up to 30 percent of older adults as their stomachs become less acidic with aging, but because B12 can be stored in the liver for three to five years, deficiency and its related cognitive damage could be developing years before signs of anemia reveal it. In this case, supplements may be a good choice.

In summary, the current evidence suggests that being folate or vitamin B12 deficient speeds up cognitive decline, and low folate may also increase the risk of Alzheimer's disease (no such relationship has been established for B12). Excessive folate may also speed up cognitive decline, especially if B12 is low. Folate naturally found in foods isn't likely to add up to high levels, but vitamin supplements and foods made with fortified grains can contribute to high folate intake.

Overall, fixing low intakes of B vitamins is the concern for cognitive decline and Alzheimer's disease, but people who are already getting enough folate and B12 through food won't necessarily benefit more from adding supplements to their diet. Future randomized clinical trials should target people with low intakes to truly test if there's a solid cause and effect.

In the meantime, natural food sources of folate, but supplement or fortified food sources of B12, are ideal. Foods that naturally provide folate include dark green vegetables like broccoli, spinach, Brussels sprouts, artichokes, and collard greens, and legumes such as edamame, chickpeas, lentils, beans, and peas. Vitamin B12 is only found naturally in animal foods such as fish and poultry, but is in some fortified milk alternatives (e.g., soy milk, rice milk, almond milk) and soy-based meat alternatives.

DID YOU KNOW?

Folate is also known as vitamin B9 but became commonly known as folate—a term related to the Latin word for leaf (folium)—in the 1940s when it was established that B9 could be found in green, leafy vegetables such as spinach, collard greens, butter lettuce, and bok choy. Today, we know that in addition to leafy greens, legumes are also a consistent source of folate, especially lentils, beans, and peas.

Flavonoids and Carotenoids

The brain is a busy place, and all that metabolic activity puts it at risk for oxidative stress and tissue damage. Antioxidant enzymes in the body are not as available to the brain as antioxidant nutrients from food, making them especially important to the aging brain. The antioxidant vitamin E was discussed at length earlier, but there are two additional classes of antioxidants that may help: carotenoids and flavonoids. The MIND diet provides plenty of flavonoids and carotenoids, especially from leafy greens and berries.

Flavonoids are biologically active polyphenolic compounds important to good health that occur naturally in a wide range of plant foods, including fruit, vegetables, chocolate, nuts, wine, and tea. There are six major subclasses of flavonoids: anthocyanidins, flavan-3-ols, flavonols, flavones, flavanones, and isoflavones. They are studied for health benefits related to cardiovascular disease, glycemic control and diabetes, certain cancers, and cognitive function (data currently limited). Major sources of flavonoids include berries such as blueberries, strawberries, raspberries, elderberries, and European black currants; vegetables such as eggplant and purple cabbage; beans such as garbanzo beans; whole grains like quinoa; and other foods such as black, green, and oolong tea, oranges, grapefruit, lemons, onions, bananas, tomatoes, and parsley.

Carotenoids are naturally occurring yellow/green, orange, and red pigments made by plants, many of which have antioxidant properties. The most common carotenoids in the American diet are alpha-carotene, beta-carotene, lycopene, lutein, zeaxanthin, and beta-cryptoxanthin. Eating carotenoid foods is linked to a reduced risk of cardiovascular disease, some cancers, age-related macular degeneration, and cataracts. Carotenoids are best absorbed with fat, such as olive oil.

Top sources of carotenoids include:

- Leafy greens such as spinach, kale, and collard greens

- Vegetables such as carrots, sweet potato, red bell pepper, pumpkin, Brussels sprouts, and broccoli

- Nuts such as pistachios

- Other fruits such as apricots, cantaloupe, oranges, watermelon, and tomatoes

There are no specific recommendations for flavonoids or carotenoids (other than the carotenoids that contribute to total vitamin A intake), and the best way to ensure adequate intake is to eat a variety of plant foods, including various vegetables, nuts, whole grains, beans, and fruit.

PART TWO
Your MIND Diet Plan

The MIND diet does nobody any good unless it is put into practice. This section of the book helps you create your own MIND diet plan. As a reminder, the MIND diet has 15 components: 10 types of food to eat and five to avoid, for a total possible weekly score of 15 for the perfect MIND diet. Points are awarded for eating the right amounts of the good foods and successfully avoiding unhealthy foods.

CHAPTER 6

What to Eat (& Avoid)

For reference, the top-scoring participants in the MIND studies ate about 1,800 calories per day, but your individual needs may be higher or lower depending on physical activity and weight management goals. It's best to work with a registered dietitian nutritionist on individual plans to meet individual needs. The Eat List on the following page details the MIND guidelines to get you started.

THE EAT LIST: WHAT TO EAT ON THE MIND DIET

Serving sizes	• Vegetables: 1 cup fresh leafy greens, ½ cup cooked leafy greens, ½ cup other vegetables • Whole grains: ½ cup cooked • Nuts: 1 ounce (about ¼ cup) • Beans: ½ cup cooked • Berries: ½ cup fresh, ¼ cup dried • Poultry: 3 ounces cooked (about 4 to 5 ounces raw) • Fish: 3 ounces cooked (about 4 to 5 ounces raw) • Olive oil: 1 tablespoon • Wine: 5 ounces
Everyday	• 3 servings of whole grains • 1 serving of vegetables (non-leafy greens) • 1 glass of wine • Olive oil
6 days a week	• 1 serving of leafy greens
5 days a week	• 1 serving of nuts
Every other day (4 days/week)	• 1 serving of beans
Twice a week	• 1 serving of berries • 1 serving of poultry (not fried)
Once a week	• 1 serving of fish (not fried)

Avoid foods on the Avoid List (below) as much as possible. If zero tolerance is not practical, aim to limit these foods according to the following guidelines. The more you can avoid these foods altogether, the better.

THE AVOID LIST: WHAT TO LIMIT ON THE MIND DIET	
Serving sizes	• Butter or margarine: 1 tablespoon • Pastries and sweets: 1 to 5 ounces (check the label), below are some examples: —Cookies: 2 pieces (1 ounce) —Light/medium cakes (e.g., coffee cake, doughnuts, angel food cake): 1 medium doughnut (2 to 3 ounces) —Heavy cakes (e.g., cheesecake, pie): 1 slice (4 to 5 ounces) • Ice cream: ½ cup • Red meat: 3 ounces cooked (about 4 to 5 ounces raw) • Whole-fat cheese: 1 ounce • Fried fast food: Any (e.g., 1 medium order of French fries)
Avoid daily	• 1 serving of butter or margarine
Avoid most days (5 days/week)	• 1 serving of pastries or sweets
Avoid most days (4 days/week)	• 1 serving of red meat
Avoid weekly (1 day/week)	For cheese and fried fast food, the recommendation is to limit to less than once a week, so if they are consumed one week, the next week would have to eliminate them completely. • 1 serving of fried fast food • 1 serving of whole-fat cheese

Keeping Score

Before even getting started with the MIND diet, it would be interesting to score your current diet for a week based on the MIND model. This will provide a baseline, and you can track progress from this point. This may be enough to help you make changes in the right direction. Start tracking your diet using the MIND Diet Weekly Scorecard, and if you'd like more detailed help, go on to the menu-planning worksheets.

A simple way to track your weekly progress is to make check marks for every serving of MIND foods—from all 15 groups—that you've eaten/avoided each meal. At the end of the week, tally your score and see how you fared. Remember that in the MIND studies, those who scored in the top two tiers were not perfect. Tier one scored 12.5 to 8.5 and tier two scored 7 to 8 points, and both were linked to brain health benefits.

MIND Diet Weekly Scorecard

There are two methods you may use for scoring yourself. Remember that the highest possible score in any category is 1, regardless of whether you use Method 1 or 2. A few things to keep in mind as you score:

- The weekly scores for whole grains and butter need to be converted to average daily scores. To do this, simply divide total weekly servings by seven.

- The score for wine is based on a strict one 5-ounce glass per day. If there is more than one glass per day, the score is 0. The score is also 0 for no wine. Points for wine are only awarded for one glass per day, no less, no more.

- For olive oil, there is no amount recommended; the score is based on if olive oil is used as the main oil or not. For simplicity's sake, a 1-serving-per-day recommendation has been added.

Method 1: Simple

Find your simple score by taking a pass/fail approach to whether or not you've followed the MIND diet for the week. This method is quicker, but is a rough estimate.

1. Enter number of servings accomplished per food group, by day.

2. To answer "did you meet targets"—Give yourself 1 point for every Y or 0 for every N.

3. Add up the total score and compare to MIND targets. (Aim for a score of 10 to 15, but remember, even scores from 7 to 8 saw some benefits. Top scorers from the research had MIND diet scores in the 8.5 to 12.5 range).

Method 2: Detailed

Calculate your detailed score by comparing your servings of food groups to the goals. This will be more accurate.

1. Give yourself 1 point for every Y.

2. For each N score, use the "detailed scoring guide" to find where your weekly total or average daily score (for whole grains and butter) fits in, then award yourself 0 or 0.5 point in the detailed score column. For each Y score, award yourself 1 point.

3. Add up the total score and compare to MIND targets. (Aim for a score of 10 to 15, but remember, even scores from 7 to 8 saw some benefits. Top scorers from the research had MIND diet scores in the 8.5 to 12.5 range.)

		MIND targets servings per week
BRAIN-HEALTHY FOODS	Whole grains	21 (3 per day)
	Other vegetables	7 (1 per day)
	Leafy greens	6
	Nuts	5
	Beans	3
	Berries	2
	Poultry	2
	Fish	1
	Wine	7 (1 per day)
	Olive oil	7 (1 per day)
BRAIN-HARMFUL FOODS	Butter	<7 tablespoons
	Pastries, Baked Goods, Sweets	<5
	Red meat	<4
	Cheese	<1
	Fried/fast food	<1

SAMPLE MIND DIET WEEKLY SCORECARD			
Week of:	*Sun*	*Mon*	*Tue*
Whole grains	3	3	2
Leafy greens	0	2	1
Other vegetables	1	1	1
Nuts	0	1	1
Beans	2	0	0
Berries	0	0	1
Poultry	0	0	0
Fish	1	0	0
Wine	1	1	1
Olive oil	1	1	1
Butter	0	0	2
Pastries, baked goods, sweets	0	0	0
Red meat	0	0	0
Whole-fat cheese	1	0	0
Fried/fast food	0	0	0

	SAMPLE MIND DIET WEEKLY SCORECARD			
Wed	Thu	Fri	Sat	Week **TOTAL**
4	1	2	0	15; 15/7=2.1
0	1	2	0	6
1	1	1	1	7
1	1	1	0	5
0	0	0	0	2
0	0	1	0	2
1	0	0	1	2
0	1	0	2	4
0	0	0	0	3
1	1	1	1	7 (1/d)
0	0	4	2	8
0	0	0	0	<5
0	0	1	2	3
0	0	1	1	3
1	0	0	0	1

WEEKLY TOTALS AND SCORE SAMPLE

	Weekly MIND Target (daily average)	Did you meet MIND targets? (Y/N)	Simple Score (0 or 1)	Detailed Score (0, 0.5, or 1)	Detailed Scoring Guide
Whole grains	21 (3/d)	N	0	0.5	0–1 = 0 1–2 = .5 3+ = 1
Leafy greens	6	Y	1	1	0–2 = 0 3–5 = .5 6+ = 1
Other vegetables	7	Y	1	1	0–4 = 0 5–6 = .5 7+ = 1
Nuts	5	Y	1	1	0–.25 = 0 .25–4 = 0.5 5+ = 1
Beans	4	N	0	1	0 = 0 1–3 = 0.5 4+ = 1
Berries	2	Y	1	1	0 = 0 1 = 0.5 2+ = 1
Poultry	2	Y	1	1	0 = 0 1 = 0.5 2+ = 1
Fish	1	Y	1	1	0 = 0 .25–.75 = 0.5 1+ = 1
Wine	7 (1/d)	N	0	0.5	0 or >1/d = 0 1/month to 6/wk = 0.5 1/d = 1

	Weekly MIND Target (daily average)	Did you meet MIND targets? (Y/N)	Simple Score (0 or 1)	Detailed Score (0, 0.5, or 1)	Detailed Scoring Guide
Olive oil	7 (1/d)	Y	1	1	not used = 0 not used = 0.5 primary oil used = 1
Butter	<7/week (<1T/d)	N	0	0.5	>2 T/d = 0 1–2 T/d = 0.5 0–0.99/d = 1
Pastries, baked goods, sweets	<5	Y	1	1	7+ = 0 5–6 = 0.5 0–4 = 1
Red meat	<4	Y	1	1	7+ = 0 4–6 = 0.5 1 = 0–3
Whole-fat cheese	<1	N	0	0.5	7+ = 0 1–6 = 0.5 0–0.99 = 1
Fried/fast food	<1	N	0	0.5	4+ = 0 1–3 = 0.5 0–0.99 = 1
Total Points:			9	12	
Your score as % (Total Points/15)			60%	80%	

TOTALS: Aim for a score of 10 to 15, but remember, even scores from 7 to 8 saw some benefits. Top scorers from the research had MIND diet scores in the 8.5 to 12.5 range.

MIND DIET WEEKLY SCORECARD

Week of:	Sun	Mon	Tue
Whole grains			
Leafy greens			
Other vegetables			
Nuts			
Beans			
Berries			
Poultry			
Fish			
Wine			
Olive oil			
Butter			
Pastries, baked goods, sweets			
Red meat			
Cheese			
Fried/fast food			

MIND DIET WEEKLY SCORECARD				
Wed	Thu	Fri	Sat	Week **TOTAL**

	Weekly MIND Target (daily average)	Did you meet MIND targets? (Y/N)	Simple Score (0 or 1)	Detailed Score (0, 0.5, or 1)	Detailed Scoring Guide
WEEKLY TOTALS AND SCORE					
Whole grains					0–1 = 0 1–2 = .5 3+ = 1
Leafy greens					0–2 = 0 3–5 = .5 6+ = 1
Other vegetables					0–4 = 0 5–6 = .5 7+ = 1
Nuts					0–.25 = 0 .25–4 = 0.5 5+ = 1
Beans					0 = 0 1–3 = 0.5 4+ = 1
Berries					0 = 0 1 = 0.5 2+ = 1
Poultry					0 = 0 1 = 0.5 2+ = 1
Fish					0 = 0 .25–.75 = 0.5 1+ = 1
Wine					0 or >1/d = 0 1/month to 6/wk = 0.5 1/d = 1

WEEKLY TOTALS AND SCORE

	Weekly MIND Target (daily average)	Did you meet MIND targets? (Y/N)	Simple Score (0 or 1)	Detailed Score (0, 0.5, or 1)	Detailed Scoring Guide
Olive oil					not used = 0 not used = 0.5 primary oil used = 1
Butter					>2 T/d = 0 1–2 T/d = 0.5 0–0.99/d = 1
Pastries, baked goods, sweets					7+ = 0 5–6 = 0.5 0–4 = 1
Red meat					7+ = 0 4–6 = 0.5 1 = 0–3
Whole-fat cheese					7+ = 0 1–6 = 0.5 0–0.99 = 1
Fried/fast food					4+ = 0 1–3 = 0.5 0–0.99 = 1
Total Points:					
Your score as % (Total Points/15)					

TOTALS: Aim for a score of 10 to 15, but remember, even scores from 7 to 8 saw some benefits. Top scorers from the research had MIND diet scores in the 8.5 to 12.5 range.

CHAPTER 7
Meal Planning

Meal planning is essential to implementing your MIND diet plan. With a little forethought and some helpful meal-planning tools, successfully following the MIND diet can be simple and efficient. The good news is that unlike other diets that ask you to translate grams of nutrients into food, the MIND diet is already based on real food. The researchers have laid the scientific foundation. All you have to worry about is deciding what goes on your plate, and the nutrient levels will take care of themselves.

The worksheets that follow will help organize food lists and menu ideas for the week. There are sample worksheets already filled out with examples, followed by blank templates for you to put your MIND diet into action.

Planning Your Food Choices

The below worksheet is filled out with food choices in each food group. It shows a range of options to give you some ideas. However, in real life, it is more practical to stick to some of the same foods for multiple meals to cut down on cooking time. For example, if you roast a pan of Brussels sprouts for dinner one night and have leftovers, they can be one of the vegetable servings for the following day. Or, if you make a large batch of brown rice, it could be used for a serving at lunch and two more servings at dinner to meet the daily recommended three servings.

When you fill out your own worksheet, the result should be a list of foods that fit the MIND diet guidelines as well as your personal preferences. It's also helpful because knowing what's in your mental "cupboard" of options is a natural way to start menu planning with a concrete set of options in hand. This step makes the menu planning stage much less daunting.

SERVING SIZES	
Vegetables	1 cup fresh leafy greens, ½ cup cooked leafy greens, ½ cup other vegetables
Whole grains	½ cup cooked
Nuts	1 ounce (about ¼ cup)
Beans	½ cup cooked
Berries	½ cup fresh, ¼ cup dried
Poultry	3 ounces cooked (about 4 to 5 ounces raw)
Fish	3 ounces cooked (about 4 to 5 ounces raw)
Olive oil	1 tablespoon
Wine	5 ounces
Butter or margarine	1 tablespoon
Pastries and sweets	1 to 5 ounces
Red meat	3 ounces cooked (about 4 to 5 ounces raw)
Whole-fat cheese	1 ounce
Fried fast food	1 regular order (e.g., medium order of French fries)

MIND FOODS WORKSHEET SAMPLE

Food group and servings per day/week	Sun	Mon	Tue
Whole grains (WG) (3/day)	Brown rice Whole grain barley Oats	Buckwheat Corn Farro	Bulgur Freekeh Einkorn
Vegetables (non-leafy greens) (1/day)	Broccoli	Carrots	Sweet potatoes
Leafy greens (6+/week)	Kale	Spinach	Arugula
Nuts (5+/week)	-	Pistachios	Almonds
Beans (4+/week)	Black beans	-	Pinto beans
Berries (2+/week)	-	-	Blueberries
Poultry (2+/week)	Skinless chicken breast	-	-
Fish (1+/week)	-	-	Wild salmon
Olive oil (use as primary oil)	1 tablespoon	1 tablespoon	1 tablespoon
Wine (1/day)	5 ounces chardonnay	5 ounces cabernet sauvignon	5 ounces pinot noir

MIND FOODS WORKSHEET SAMPLE			
Wed	*Thu*	*Fri*	*Sat*
Millet White quinoa Rye	Popcorn Spelt Sorghum	Whole wheat pasta Teff Wild rice	Triticale Red rice Black or red quinoa
Brussels sprouts	Green beans	Beets	Zucchini
Cabbage	Collard greens	Romaine lettuce	-
Walnuts	Pecans	Hazelnuts	-
-	Kidney beans	-	Garbanzo beans
-	-	Strawberries	-
Lean ground turkey	-	-	-
-	-	-	-
1 tablespoon	1 tablespoon	1 tablespoon	
5 ounces viognier	5 ounces rosé	5 ounces merlot	5 ounces sauvignon blanc

Avoid these foods as much as possible. Examples of allowable amounts of these foods are listed below purely for illustration. It is better if you can avoid them altogether. For cheese and fast food, the recommendation is to limit to less than once a week, so if the below foods were consumed one week, the next week would have to eliminate them completely.

MIND FOODS WORKSHEET SAMPLE			
Food group and servings per day/week	Sun	Mon	Tue
Whole-fat cheese (<1/week) Max: 0–1/wk	1 ounce cheddar cheese	-	-
Fried fast food (<1/week) Max: 0–1/wk	-	1 small order of French fries	-
Red meat (<4/week) Max: 3/wk	-	-	3 ounces steak
Pastries or sweets (<5/week) Max: 4/week	2 small cookies	1 small blueberry muffin	-
Butter or margarine (<1T/d) Max: 6.99 T/week	1 teaspoon butter	1 teaspoon butter	1 teaspoon butter

MIND FOODS WORKSHEET SAMPLE			
Wed	*Thu*	*Fri*	*Sat*
-	-	-	-
-	-	-	-
-	1 small hamburger	-	3 ounces meatballs
-	1 small croissant	-	1 small brownie
1 teaspoon butter	1 teaspoon margarine	1 teaspoon margarine	1 teaspoon margarine

Sample MIND Menu Worksheet

Use the sample MIND Menu Worksheet provided here to fill in menu ideas. Here's what a week on the MIND diet could look like. Full of healthy, whole foods, it's not just brain food, it's heart-healthy and diabetes-friendly, and provides lasting energy that will fill you up but won't slow you down thanks to the filling fiber and balance of healthy proteins and fats.

MIND MENU WORKSHEET SAMPLE			
Day	*Sun*	*Mon*	*Tues*
Breakfast	Blueberry-Coconut Overnight Oats (page 145)	Creamy Berry Smoothie (page 146)	Green Smoothie (page 147)
AM Snack	High-Protein Banana Chocolate Chip Breakfast Cookies (page 231)	½ ounce pistachios	1 ounce almonds
Lunch	Red Quinoa and Navy Bean Salad with Toasted Almonds, Cilantro, and Lime Cumin Vinaigrette (page 164)	Grab-and-Go Pita Slaw Sandwich (page 156) Fattoush Salad (page 191)	Quick Chicken-Tortilla Soup (page 203)
PM Snack	Strawberry and Baby Arugula Salad (page 187)	½ ounce pistachios	½ cup oatmeal

MIND MENU WORKSHEET SAMPLE

Wed	Thu	Fri	Sat
One-Egg Wonder (page 147)	White Bean–Tomato Toast (page 148)	Avocado Toast (page 149)	Raspberry Almond Oat Shake (page 231)
1 ounce walnuts	½ ounce pecans	½ ounce hazelnuts	Warm Rosemary Pistachios (page 223)
White Bean and Whole Grain Pasta Soup (page 208)	Mediterranean-Style Watermelon-Pistachio-Mint Couscous (page 217)	Turkey-Ginger Sliders (page 173) Kale Apple Carrot Salad (page 188)	Edamame, Amaranth, and Chimichurri Nourish Bowl (page 158)
3 cups popcorn	½ ounce pecans	½ ounce hazelnuts	Guacamole-Stuffed Tomato Poppers (page 221)

MIND MENU WORKSHEET SAMPLE			
Day	*Sun*	*Mon*	*Tues*
Dinner	Roasted Chicken with Fennel, Carrots, and Dried Plums (page 170) Oat Cranberry Pilaf with Pistachios (page 213) 5 ounces wine	Pistachio-Crusted Trout (page 180) Pomegranate Avocado Quinoa Grain Salad (page 197) 5 ounces wine	Tango Fish Tacos (page 181) Fiesta Quinoa (page 218) 5 ounces wine

Creating Your Own Meal Plans: Blank Worksheet

MIND FOODS MENU PLANNER			
Day	*Breakfast*	*AM Snack*	*Lunch*
SUNDAY			

MIND MENU WORKSHEET SAMPLE

Wed	Thu	Fri	Sat
Tango Fish Tacos (page 181) Fiesta Quinoa (page 218) 5 ounces wine	Curried Chickpea Quinoa Loaf (page 162) Butternut Squash Curry-Ginger Soup (page 207) 5 ounces wine	Almond-Crusted Baked Salmon (page 176) Mediterranean Orange Wheat (page 216) 5 ounces wine	Lentil Patties with Basil Arugula Cashew Cream (page 160) Freekeh with Blueberries (page 214) 5 ounces wine

MIND FOODS MENU PLANNER

PM Snack	Dinner	MIND foods
		Whole grains: Vegetables: Leafy greens: Nuts: Beans: Berries: Poultry: Fish: Olive oil: Wine:

MIND FOODS MENU PLANNER

Day	Breakfast	AM Snack	Lunch
MONDAY			
TUESDAY			

MIND FOODS MENU PLANNER		
PM Snack	Dinner	MIND foods
		Whole grains: Vegetables: Leafy greens: Nuts: Beans: Berries: Poultry: Fish: Olive oil: Wine:
		Whole grains: Vegetables: Leafy greens: Nuts: Beans: Berries: Poultry: Fish: Olive oil: Wine:

MIND FOODS MENU PLANNER			
Day	Breakfast	AM Snack	Lunch
WEDNESDAY			
THURSDAY			
FRIDAY			

PM Snack	Dinner	MIND foods
		Whole grains: Vegetables: Leafy greens: Nuts: Beans: Berries: Poultry: Fish: Olive oil: Wine:
		Whole grains: Vegetables: Leafy greens: Nuts: Beans: Berries: Poultry: Fish: Olive oil: Wine:
		Whole grains: Vegetables: Leafy greens: Nuts: Beans: Berries: Poultry: Fish: Olive oil: Wine:

MIND FOODS MENU PLANNER

MIND FOODS MENU PLANNER

Day	Breakfast	AM Snack	Lunch
SATURDAY			

Food Safety

Cooking is an act of caring and generosity. You want your dishes to be delicious and nourishing, but first you want to ensure that they won't make anyone sick from food safety mistakes.

Food safety—from shopping to preparation and storage— is important for everyone, but especially the very young, older adults, anyone with a compromised immune system, and anyone responsible for providing food to these groups. The risk of food poisoning is higher in these groups, and the consequences can be severe.

For these groups, it is recommended to only eat seafood, meat, poultry, or eggs that have been fully cooked to safe temperatures; avoid sprouts, raw juice, raw milk, and anything made from unpasteurized milk (e.g., this category could include Brie, Camembert, Asadero, Panela, queso blanco, queso fresco, yogurt, pudding, ice cream, and frozen yogurt, if made from unpasteurized milk—check the label); and heat up deli meats to kill listeria bacteria.

MIND FOODS MENU PLANNER		
PM Snack	Dinner	MIND foods
		Whole grains:
		Vegetables:
		Leafy greens:
		Nuts:
		Beans:
		Berries:
		Poultry:
		Fish:
		Olive oil:
		Wine:

Following are general guidelines that anyone working with food should embrace.

1. Wash hands well, and wash them often. That means washing hands with soap for at least 20 seconds. When working with food, wash hands, at a minimum, before starting to cook, after handling raw meat, and after food prep is finished. While washing up after raw meat is a must, it doesn't hurt to wash in between preparing other foods too (e.g., between chopping an onion and chopping greens), as bacteria can cross-contaminate between any foods.

2. Separate foods that could cross-contaminate each other. That means having separate cutting boards for raw meat versus fruits and vegetables, and using different knives to work with each. If that's not possible, be sure to thoroughly wash and sanitize knives before switching foods. Also, fruits and vegetables should be rinsed before coming to the cutting board to reduce the risk of transferring bacteria to the cutting board. All cutting boards and knives should be

washed well with hot water and soap after use. Old cutting boards with visible grooves (where bacteria can hide) should be replaced. Wipe down and sanitize counters and cooking areas before and after food prep.

3. Be aware of food temperatures. Keep hot foods hot (above 140°F), cold foods cold (below 40°F), and frozen foods freezing (below 0°F). Bacteria love to grow between 40°F and 140°F, and will multiply in the right conditions. Don't leave prepared food out for more than two hours. On hotter days, cut that time down to no more than an hour. Make sure your refrigerator is maintaining a temperature of 40°F or below.

4. Be aware of cooking temperatures. Raw meat, fish, and poultry must be cooked to safe temperatures. Poultry must be cooked to 165°F. Fresh seafood must be cooked to 145°F (for shellfish, cook until the flesh is opaque; for clams, mussels, and oysters, cook until their shells open). Meat needs to be cooked to 145°F, unless it is ground, which needs to reach 160°F. Food thermometers are an essential kitchen tool to confirm internal cooking temperatures.

5. There's a right way to refrigerate hot food. Store hot food in small, shallow containers, which provide more surface area to allow the food to cool down quickly and evenly, so bacteria has less chance to find a comfortable environment to grow in. The down side is that introducing hot food into the refrigerator makes the refrigerator work harder. To minimize this effect, place all the hot foods in storage containers before opening the refrigerator door, then place at the bottom back of the refrigerator (the coldest area), before quickly closing the door again.

6. Defrost food in the refrigerator or the microwave. Gone are the days when it is considered safe to defrost food on the kitchen counter.

7. Don't overstuff the refrigerator. Some space is required for cool air to flow and do its job. Taking stock of the refrigerator's contents is good policy anyway. It ensures you are regularly eating your perishable foods and that you don't keep past-due food lurking at the back of your refrigerator. At least once a week, check your refrigerator for any foods that need to be discarded.

8. Keep your sink, counters, refrigerator drawers, utensil drawers, buttons, and handles, contamination-free. Wash all these areas regularly with soap and water, and replace or sanitize kitchen sponges often, at least weekly. Soaked sponges can be microwaved for a minute or two, or run in the dishwasher with the dry heat setting, to help sanitize them. Scrub sponges can be saturated with a quarter cup of water and microwaved for a minute; cellulose sponges can be soaked in a half-cup of water and microwaved for two minutes.

9. Rinse all fruits and vegetables except those that are labeled as prewashed and ready to eat. On the other hand, do not rinse raw seafood, meat, and poultry. It turns out that rinsing can do more harm, spreading bacteria rather than washing it away.

Leafy Greens

The following tips are specifically for green, leafy vegetables, which are often eaten raw. Raw foods raise inherent food safety concerns. Leafy greens are very healthy foods, so it's worth the effort to learn the simple techniques to ensure they're safe to eat. To keep leafy greens safe, it's all about prevention and avoiding the introduction of bad bacteria—from the farm all the way up until it reaches the fork.

1. From the farm to the grocery store, your power is in choosing from trusted producers and retailers.

2. Starting at the grocery store, be sure greens are in a refrigerated area, and don't buy anything that looks wilted or brown. While shopping and when checking out, keep greens bagged and separated from raw meat and poultry.

3. Once at home, store fresh leafy greens in a clean refrigerator at 40°F or below. Don't store leafy greens near raw meat. Always keep leafy greens stored above raw meat to avoid meat juices dripping onto the greens.

4. Before and after handling fresh leafy greens, wash hands for 20 seconds with warm water and soap. Outer leaves of greens can be thrown out. Cut away any parts that look damaged or bruised.

5. Wash leafy greens thoroughly, which can help reduce bacteria that might be present, though it won't completely get rid of them. Rinse all the greens, even the small, tightly packed leaves at the center of a head of lettuce. Soak greens in cool water, agitate them gently, then let them sit for a few minutes to let any debris sink, then lift them out of the bowl into a colander (this is important since draining alone simply adds the debris back into the mix), and rinse under running water. The agitate-and-soak process can be repeated two to three times for crinkly greens (anything that's not totally flat-leafed), such as spinach, before rinsing.

6. If buying prewashed greens, confirm that it really is, as packaged greens can look alike, prewashed or not. Look for

the terms "prewashed," "triple-washed," or "ready to eat." Prewashed greens don't technically need another wash at home (and are washed in facilities that are cleaner than the average home kitchen). If you plan to wash your greens at home, it's more affordable to start with unwashed greens.

7. Cooking can also help kill harmful bacteria, which won't apply to all leafy greens, but is one way to enjoy hardier greens such as kale, collards, and spinach. Cooking for 15 seconds at 160°F is all it takes to ensure these greens are safe.

8. Keep in mind that local and organically grown greens aren't necessarily any safer, and they should be washed with just as much care. There are antimicrobial produce washes on the market, but there's no proof they are any more effective than regular washing at home. This may change as better produce washes are developed for both commercial and home use.

Stocking Your Kitchen

A well-stocked pantry is the foundation to any meal. Keep healthy staples on hand, and a nourishing meal will always be in reach. For items in cans or boxes, look for BPA-free cans or aseptic packaging.

Dry Pantry

Vegetables: Corn, garlic, onions, potatoes, tomatoes (whole, diced, crushed, pureed, or made into a paste), roasted red peppers
Nuts: Almonds (whole, sliced, butter, milk), pistachios, walnuts
Beans: Black, cannellini, chickpeas, great northern, navy, pinto, red kidney
Fish: Tuna, anchovy fillets or paste

Whole grains: Barley, brown rice, bulgur, farro, pasta (whole grain, assorted shapes), popping corn, quinoa, steel-cut oats, wild rice

Oil: Extra-virgin olive oil, grapeseed oil

Wine: Red (cabernet sauvignon, pinot noir), white (chardonnay, Riesling, sauvignon blanc)

Other: Herbs and spices (chili powder, crushed red pepper, curry powder, cinnamon, cumin, ginger, oregano, pepper, rosemary, salt, thyme)

Other: Vinegars (distilled, apple cider, red wine, rice wine, champagne, balsamic)

Other: Capers or olives, lentils, low-sodium vegetable broth, low-sodium chicken broth, coffee, tea

Freezer

Vegetables: Broccoli, carrots, edamame, green beans, peas

Leafy greens: Kale, spinach

Nuts: Almonds, pistachios, walnuts

Berries: Blueberries, raspberries, strawberries

Poultry: Boneless, skinless chicken breasts, ground turkey

Fish: Salmon, shrimp

Whole grains: Corn, red rice

Refrigerator

Vegetables: Bell peppers, broccoli, carrots, cauliflower, celery, garlic, ginger root, onions, tomatoes

Leafy greens: Arugula, chard, kale, spinach

Other: Hot sauce, lemons, mustard (Dijon, whole grain), soy sauce

PART THREE
Recipes

The MIND diet is simple. There are no calories to count or long lists of foods to avoid. The eating pattern is based on food, not specific nutrients or overly prescriptive diet rules. This is about everyday eating. Simply follow the basic guidelines of the MIND diet—eat from the 10 basic brain-healthy food groups, avoid the five brain-harming ones—and rest assured that there's a body of current science that supports its role in brain health and overall nourishment.

To get you started, this chapter features 75 recipes. More than 25 of the nation's top nutrition experts—all registered dietitians—who love good eating and healthy living in equal measure, share their favorite recipes. Each recipe has nutrition information per serving and lists which MIND foods are included, so it's easy to see what food groups are accounted for.

Many of these recipes have a Mediterranean flare, as they're a natural fit for the MIND diet. However, that doesn't mean other culinary traditions can't fit into the MIND diet—from tacos to sriracha-spiced entrées, there are plenty of choices in between. The MIND diet foods are versatile and can fit just about any cuisine your palate is craving.

Breakfast

Blueberry-Coconut Overnight Oats

These easy, flavorful Blueberry-Coconut Overnight Oats are the perfect make-ahead healthy breakfast treat. They take just a few minutes to prepare, then they "cook" in the refrigerator overnight. This recipe has protein and calcium from Greek yogurt, fiber from healthy whole grain oats, and natural sweetness from fruit and coconut. Find this simple, beautiful breakfast ready and waiting in the refrigerator when you wake up in the morning.

MIND foods: Berries, whole grains

Yield: 2 servings

Time: 5 minutes to prep; 5+ hours refrigeration

Difficulty: Easy

> ¾ cup frozen blueberries
>
> ½ banana
>
> ¾ cup plain Greek yogurt
>
> ½ cup water
>
> ¾ cup rolled oats
>
> 3 tablespoons unsweetened shredded coconut

1. Place blueberries, banana, yogurt, and water in a blender and blend until smooth. Pour the blueberry mixture into a bowl. Mix in the oats and coconut. Separate the mixture into two containers or jars, cover, and refrigerate for at least 5 hours or overnight.

Nutrition: 270 calories, 5 g total fat, 3 g saturated fat, 15 g protein, 43 g carbohydrates, 6 g fiber

Recipe by Amber Ketchum, MDS, RD | www.homemadenutrition.com

Creamy Berry Smoothie

This superfood smoothie features the berries most researched for brain health: blueberries and strawberries. A protein bonus comes from the almond butter and soft tofu, a mild-tasting and very blendable kind of tofu that incorporates seamlessly into soups and smoothies, where it adds a high-protein, vegetarian, and dairy-free creaminess.

MIND foods: Berries, nuts, beans

Yield: 2 servings

Time: 5 minutes

Difficulty: Easy

   1 cup fresh or frozen strawberries

   1 cup fresh or frozen blueberries

   ½ cup soft tofu, drained

   1 tablespoon almond butter

   ½ cup unsweetened almond-coconut milk blend

   1 ice cube (optional)

1. Combine all ingredients in a blender. Pulse until fully combined. Additional ice cubes may be added for a colder temperature or thinner consistency, according to preference.

Nutrition: 180 calories, 8 g total fat, 1 g saturated fat, 6 g protein, 24 g carbohydrates, 5 g fiber

Green Smoothie

This green smoothie is a refreshing way to add more leafy greens into the day's diet.

MIND foods: Berries, leafy greens

Yield: 1 serving

Time: 5 minutes

Difficulty: Easy

> *1 cup fresh or frozen blueberries*
>
> *1 cup fresh or ½ cup frozen baby spinach*
>
> *1 cup almond milk*
>
> *1 tablespoon chia seeds*

1. Combine all ingredients in a blender. Pulse until smooth.

Nutrition: 210 calories, 8 g total fat, 1 g saturated fat, 5 g protein, 33 g carbohydrates, 11 g fiber

One-Egg Wonder

This super-simple breakfast is quick and easy to prepare, perfect for days when there just isn't a lot of time to spend on breakfast.

MIND foods: Vegetables, olive oil

Yield: 1 serving

Time: 3 minutes

Difficulty: Easy

> *1 egg*
>
> *3 heirloom cherry tomatoes, halved*
>
> *1 teaspoon extra-virgin olive oil*
>
> *Salt and pepper, to taste*

1. Into a 4- to 6-ounce ramekin, crack the egg. Beat the egg with a fork to incorporate a lot of air, which will result in a fluffier cooked egg. Microwave for 45 to 60 seconds. Carefully remove from microwave as the ramekin will be hot. Top with tomato halves and drizzle with olive oil. Sprinkle with fresh pepper and salt. Enjoy.

Nutrition: 120 calories, 10 g total fat, 2 g saturated fat, 7 g protein, 2 g carbohydrates, 1 g fiber

White Bean–Tomato Toast

Breakfast can be quick and simple. This recipe will have you energized and ready for your day in no time.

MIND foods: Whole grains, beans, olive oil

Yield: 1 serving

Time: 5 minutes

Difficulty: Easy

    1 slice 100% whole wheat bread

    1 (15-ounce) can white beans, drained and rinsed

    4 teaspoons extra-virgin olive oil, divided

    1 lemon, juiced

    Salt and pepper, to taste

    5 cherry tomatoes, halved

1. Place bread in a toaster. Meanwhile, blend beans, 3 teaspoons of olive oil, lemon juice, and salt and pepper until uniform. It should have a spread-like consistency, similar to hummus. If needed, add more olive oil until desired consistency is reached. Spread 2 tablespoons of the white bean mixture onto the toast, top with halved tomatoes, and drizzle with remaining teaspoon of olive oil.

2. Season with additional pepper, as desired. There will be leftover spread, which can be refrigerated and enjoyed for up to five days. This recipe can be repeated, or the spread can be enjoyed as a dip in an easy snack with strips of carrots, celery, cucumbers, or bell peppers.

Nutrition: 200 calories, 8 g total fat, 1 g saturated fat, 8 g protein, 27 g carbohydrates, 6 g fiber

Avocado Toast

Making avocado the centerpiece of any meal is a recipe for indulgence and good health due to its healthy unsaturated fats. California avocados are best because of ideal growing practices and consistent high-quality fruit. Red onions, chili pepper flakes, and lemon juice add complementary bright notes.

MIND foods: Whole grains, olive oil

Yield: 4 servings

Time: 5 minutes

Difficulty: Easy

> *4 slices 100% whole wheat bread*
>
> *1 small avocado, peeled, deseeded, and mashed*
>
> *½ small red onion, thinly sliced*
>
> *2 teaspoons extra-virgin olive oil*
>
> *½ teaspoon chili pepper flakes*
>
> *Salt and pepper, to taste*
>
> *1 lemon, quartered*

1. Toast bread to desired doneness. Evenly distributing among four slices of toast, spread the mashed avocado, top with red onion slices, drizzle with olive oil, and sprinkle with chili pepper flakes and salt and pepper. Serve each slice of toast with a quarter of a lemon, to be squeezed over toast just before eating.

Nutrition: 150 calories, 8 g total fat, 1 g saturated fat, 4 g protein, 16 g carbohydrates, 4 g fiber

Winter Frittata

This Winter Frittata features healthy comfort foods like dark orange or purple sweet potatoes, Brussels sprouts, and earthy onions.

MIND foods: Vegetables, olive oil

Yield: 6 servings

Time: 15 minutes to prep; 1 hour 5 minutes to cook

Difficulty: Easy

> 2 cups diced sweet potatoes, such as purple Okinawan sweet potatoes
>
> 1 cup quartered Brussels sprouts
>
> 1 cup roughly chopped yellow onions
>
> 6 garlic cloves, minced
>
> ¼ cup fresh chopped rosemary, divided
>
> 2 tablespoons extra-virgin olive oil, divided
>
> Salt and pepper, to taste
>
> 6 eggs

1. Preheat the oven to 400°F. In a large bowl, combine potatoes, Brussels sprouts, onions, garlic, half of the rosemary, 1 tablespoon of the olive oil, and salt and pepper (ideally, no more than a small pinch of salt).

2. Mix until all of the potatoes and Brussels sprouts are evenly coated. It's easiest to do this by hand, and disposable plastic kitchen gloves keep the mess to a minimum. Transfer the bowl's contents onto a large sheet pan in one even layer and roast in the oven for 45 minutes or until potatoes are fully cooked (to test, pick a potato piece from the center of the baking sheet, allow to cool enough to allow you to taste for doneness).

3. Meanwhile, in a medium bowl, lightly whisk eggs until uniform, then add salt and pepper. Set aside. When potato–Brussels sprouts mixture is nearly finished roasting, heat remaining

tablespoon of olive oil in a 12–inch, oven-safe skillet over medium heat, then add potato-Brussels sprouts mixture from oven to skillet, pour eggs into the skillet, and stir to combine.

4. Reduce oven heat to 350°F. Cook skillet contents for 4 to 5 minutes to allow the egg to start setting; the edges will start to pull away from the pan. Top with remaining rosemary. Place pan into oven and bake for 15 minutes or until set. Let rest 2 minutes before serving. To cut down on cooking time, the roasted vegetables can be made a day in advance. Another option is to use up any kind of leftover roasted vegetables from a previous meal with this simple frittata recipe.

Nutrition: 190 calories, 10 g total fat, 2 g saturated fat, 8 g protein, 18 g carbohydrates, 4 g fiber

Spring Frittata

This Spring Frittata celebrates eggs, an affordable and quick-cooking protein for easy meals. A frittata is a simple way to pull together a meal for breakfast, lunch, or dinner that tastes just as good hot as it does room temperature or even cold.

MIND foods: Nuts, olive oil, vegetables

Yield: 6 servings

Time: 10 minutes to prep; 20 minutes to cook

Difficulty: Easy

¼ cup almond slices

6 eggs, beaten

¼ cup sliced green onions bulbs (white parts)

½ teaspoon pepper

Pinch salt

1 tablespoon extra-virgin olive oil

½ cup asparagus, chopped into about 1-inch pieces

1 tablespoon chopped fresh flat-leaf parsley

2 tablespoons sliced green onion stems (green parts), for garnish (optional)

1. Preheat the oven to 350°F. In a small dry skillet, toast almond slices over medium heat, stirring frequently until fragrant and color begins to show. Do not let almonds get too brown or burn. Set aside.

2. In a medium bowl, lightly whisk the eggs until uniform, then add the sliced green onion bulbs, pepper, and salt. Set aside.

3. Heat olive oil in a 12-inch, oven-safe skillet over medium heat then sauté asparagus until fragrant, 3 to 4 minutes. Pour egg mixture into pan and stir. Cook for 4 to 5 minutes to allow the egg to start setting; the edges will start to pull away from the pan. Top with parsley, almond slices, and green onion stems. Place pan into oven and bake for 15 minutes or until set. Let rest 2 minutes before serving.

Nutrition: 130 calories, 10 g total fat, 2 g saturated fat, 8 g protein, 2 g carbohydrates, 1 g fiber

Summer Frittata

Summer smells like basil and tastes like sweet corn, which means this frittata is going to be a seasonal favorite.

MIND foods: Olive oil, vegetables, poultry

Yield: 6 servings

Time: 10 minutes to prep; 30 minutes to cook

Difficulty: Easy

    6 eggs

    Salt and pepper, to taste

    4 teaspoons extra-virgin olive oil, divided

½ small yellow onion, thinly sliced

½ cup shredded zucchini

½ cup fresh, frozen, or canned sweet corn

1 medium red bell pepper, cored, seeds removed, and diced

1 cup cooked chicken breast, shredded

2 tablespoons chopped fresh basil divided

6 small basil leaves, for garnish (optional)

1. Preheat the oven to 350°F. In a medium bowl, lightly whisk the eggs until uniform, then add salt and pepper. Set aside. Heat 2 teaspoons of the olive oil in a 12-inch, oven-safe skillet over medium heat then sauté the onion, zucchini, sweet corn, and bell pepper until fragrant and wilted, 3 to 5 minutes. Remove from heat and transfer to a colander where excess liquid may drain; gently press on vegetables with a wooden spoon to assist draining.

2. Meanwhile, bring the now-empty skillet back to the stove, and heat 2 teaspoons of remaining olive oil over medium heat. Add the chicken and half the chopped basil, and sauté until just combined, 1 to 2 minutes. Add the drained mixed vegetables and stir to combine for another minute.

3. Pour egg mixture and remaining chopped basil into the pan and stir gently. Cook for 4 to 5 minutes to allow the egg to start setting; the edges will start to pull away from the pan. Place pan into oven and bake for 15 minutes or until set. Let rest 2 minutes before serving. If desired, garnish with basil leaves.

Nutrition: 180 calories, 9 g total fat, 2 g saturated fat, 15 g protein, 8 g carbohydrates, 1 g fiber

Fall Frittata

This hearty frittata combines the warm and earthy flavors of kale and mushrooms with mild white beans.

MIND foods: Olive oil, leafy greens, vegetables, beans

Yield: 6 servings

Time: 10 minutes to prep; 30 minutes to cook

Difficulty: Easy

> 6 eggs
>
> 1 tablespoon extra-virgin olive oil
>
> ½ small yellow onion, thinly sliced
>
> 1 bunch lacinato kale, chopped
>
> 4 ounces baby portabello mushrooms, sliced
>
> 1 cup canned white beans, drained and rinsed
>
> 1 teaspoon dried sage
>
> 1 small lemon to squeeze over finished dish (optional)
>
> Salt and pepper

1. Preheat the oven to 350°F. In a medium bowl, lightly whisk the eggs until uniform, then add salt and pepper, to taste. Set aside. Heat olive oil in a 12-inch, oven-safe skillet over medium heat then sauté onion until fragrant, 2 to 3 minutes. Add kale and mushrooms, and sauté until wilted, 3 to 5 minutes. Add beans, sprinkle with sage and a pinch of salt and pepper. Stir all ingredients well, until beans are heated through, 2 to 3 minutes.

2. Pour egg mixture into pan and stir gently. Cook for 4 to 5 minutes to allow the egg to start setting; the edges will start to pull away from the pan. Place pan into oven and bake for 15 minutes or until set. Let rest 2 minutes before serving. If desired, squeeze fresh lemon juice over the final product before enjoying.

Nutrition: 140 calories, 7 g total fat, 2 g saturated fat, 10 g protein, 9 g carbohydrates, 2 g fiber

Broiled Heirloom Tomato and Rosemary Frittata

In a variation on the theme of baked frittatas, this version utilizes a smaller pan, smaller batch, and the broiler for quick cooking. It's perfect for an intimate brunch or when you want a quick meal for one, plus leftovers.

MIND foods: Olive oil, vegetables

Yield: 2 servings

Time: 10 minutes to prep; 30 minutes to cook

Difficulty: Easy

> 1 tablespoon extra-virgin olive oil
>
> ½ small yellow onion, diced
>
> ½ cup quartered heirloom cherry tomatoes
>
> 1 tablespoon chopped fresh rosemary, divided
>
> 4 eggs, whisked
>
> Salt and pepper (optional)

1. Preheat the oven broiler. In an oven-safe, 8-inch pan, heat olive oil over low-medium heat. Add onion and sauté until fragrant, 1 to 2 minutes. Add cherry tomatoes until warmed through and liquid begins to simmer, 2 to 3 minutes. Sprinkle with salt and pepper, if desired. Add most of the rosemary and stir for another minute (any remaining rosemary will be used for garnish).

2. Pour eggs into pan and quickly and gently stir to evenly distribute ingredients. Let sit, cooking until bubbles reach the surface and the edges begin to pull away from pan. Turn off heat.

3. Top with remaining rosemary and a final dash of salt and pepper, if desired. Transfer pan to broiler for 1 to 2 minutes until top is lightly browned. Remove from broiler and let cool for 1 to 2 minutes before serving.

Nutrition: 280 calories, 17 g total fat, 4 g saturated fat, 14 g protein, 8 g carbohydrates, 2 g fiber

Mains

Grab-and-Go Pita Slaw Sandwich

This sandwich is a cinch to throw together and perfect after a long day if you don't have much time to cook. It's also an easy way to get your veggies in if you want a quick, healthy lunch. If you're hungry and want something crunchy and satisfying, you've found your match. And if you want an easy sandwich for your kid's lunch box, simply make this and then slice a hard-boiled egg, put it in foil, and let them add it to their sandwich at lunchtime.

MIND foods: Whole grains, leafy greens, vegetables, beans

Yield: 2 sandwiches

Time: 5 minutes (add 15 minutes if hard-boiling an egg)

Difficulty: Easy

> 1 whole wheat pita
>
> 2 cups mixed greens, romaine lettuce, or broccoli slaw
>
> 2 teaspoons chopped jalapeño or green bell pepper
>
> 4 pieces sun-dried tomato
>
> 2 tablespoons store-bought hummus
>
> 1 hard-boiled egg (optional)

1. Cut pita in half and place in toaster if you like it slightly crunchy. Add 1 cup of lettuce mix and 1 teaspoon of jalapeño or green bell pepper to each pita half. Add 2 pieces of sun-dried tomatoes, 1 tablespoon of hummus, and half of the hard-boiled

egg (if desired) to each half. Wrap up in foil or a Ziploc bag and take on the go!

Tip: If making the hard-boiled egg, add egg to cool water in a small pot and bring up to a boil, then turn off heat, cover, and let rest for 12 minutes before removing from hot water, rinsing in an ice bath, and peeling.

Try using prewashed broccoli slaw for this recipe. It looks like shredded carrots, only it's green, and you can find it in the produce section of most stores. It's one of the best inventions to make our lives easier and our food tasty.

Nutrition: 190 calories, 5 g total fat, 1 g saturated fat, 11 g protein, 28 g carbohydrates, 6 g fiber.

Recipe by Lyssie Lakatos and Tammy Lakatos Shames, RD, CDN, CFT, aka The Nutrition Twins® | www.nutritiontwins.com

Lime Curry Avocado Egg Salad Sandwich

This recipe is a simple and fast lunch to whip up. It incorporates heart-healthy fats from avocado and is jam-packed with high-quality protein, as well as anti-inflammatory benefits from the curry (i.e., from the curcumin in turmeric and vitamin C in the fresh lime juice).

MIND foods: Whole grains

Yield: 1 sandwich

Time: 15 minutes

Difficulty: Easy

1 hard-boiled egg, diced

¼ avocado, diced

1 scallion, thinly sliced

½ fresh lime, squeezed

½ teaspoon curry powder

Pinch salt

1 whole wheat English muffin, toasted

1. To hard-boil the egg, place it in a pot and fill with water until egg is just covered. Bring to a rolling boil, turn off heat, cover, and allow egg to sit in the hot water for 10 minutes. Once time is up, drain and give egg an ice bath. Roll the cooled egg on the countertop to crack shell and allow it to come off smoothly.

2. While the egg cooks, add the avocado, scallion, lime juice, curry powder, and salt to a small mixing bowl to combine. Add egg and gently toss until well-blended. Spoon salad onto half of the English muffin and top with the other half.

Nutrition: 310 calories, 14 g total fat, 3 g saturated fat, 14 g protein, 37 g carbohydrates, 10 g fiber

Recipe by Vicki Shanta Retelny, RDN, LDN | www.simplecravingsrealfood.com

Edamame, Amaranth, and Chimichurri Nourish Bowl

A nourish bowl is a perfectly well-balanced and complete meal in one dish. This huge salad contains lots of colorful vegetables, dark leafy greens, fiber-filled whole grains, heart-healthy fat (olive oil), and plant-based protein (edamame, amaranth). You will definitely enjoy it. It's a bundle of love and nutrition in one. Cheers to your vitality, taste buds, and happiness.

MIND foods: Vegetables, leafy greens, beans, whole grains, olive oil

Yield: 4 servings

Time: 8 minutes to prep; 20 minutes to cook

Difficulty: Easy

2½ cups water

1 tablespoon loose vegetable bouillon

1 cup amaranth

1 zucchini, sliced in rounds

1 small head cauliflower, chopped into florets

1 small red onion, slivered

1 red bell pepper, deseeded and sliced into 12 big chunks

Cooking spray

2 cups edamame, shelled

1 bunch spinach, chopped

1 carrot, grated

Chimichurri Dressing:

1 bunch cilantro

1 lemon, juiced

1 clove garlic

1 tablespoon extra-virgin olive oil

Salt, to taste

1. Preheat the oven to 400°F. In a medium pot, bring the water and bouillon to a boil. Add the amaranth and cook for 20 minutes until the water is absorbed.

2. While the amaranth is cooking, make the Chimichurri Dressing. Puree the cilantro, lemon juice, garlic, olive oil, and salt in a food processor. The dressing will be thick.

3. In a medium bowl, toss half of the cilantro puree with the zucchini, cauliflower, red onion, and red pepper. Spray a roasting pan with cooking spray and add the tossed vegetables to the pan. Roast the vegetables for 20 minutes.

4. When the amaranth and roasted vegetables are done cooking, remove them from the stovetop and oven. In a large bowl, mix

together the cooked amaranth, roasted vegetables, edamame, spinach, and carrot with the chimichurri dressing. Serve.

Nutrition: 370 calories, 11 g total fat, 2 g saturated fat, 19 g protein, 54 g carbohydrates, 13 g fiber

Recipe by Sarah Koszyk, MA, RDN | www.sarahkoszyk.com

Lentil Patties with Basil Arugula Cashew Cream

These crowd-pleasing lentil patties are so easy to whip up. Served with creamy, herb-cashew cream, they also look elegant enough to offer at any dinner party. These patties are also excellent as leftovers, or even as veggie burgers on whole grain buns with the Basil Arugula Cashew Cream as a spread.

MIND foods: Vegetables, leafy greens, nuts, whole grains, olive oil

Yield: 10 patties and 12 cashew cream servings

Time: 3 hours 5 minutes to make cashew cream; 15 minutes to prep; 1 hour 15 minutes to cook

Difficulty: Medium

Lentil Patties:

1 cup uncooked small green lentils

3 cups vegetable broth

1 tablespoon chia seeds

2 medium carrots, shredded finely

1 medium yellow potato, shredded finely

4 green onions, chopped finely

¼ cup arugula, chopped finely

2 tablespoons finely chopped basil

1 clove garlic, minced

1 teaspoon Dijon mustard

½ cup dry old-fashioned oats

⅓ cup whole grain breadcrumbs

1 teaspoon soy sauce

Sea salt and pepper, to taste (optional)

2 tablespoons extra-virgin olive oil, divided

Basil Arugula Cashew Cream:

2 cups cashews

1 cup water, plus more for soaking

1 small lemon, juiced

2 tablespoons fresh arugula

2 tablespoons fresh basil

1. Place lentils in a small pot and add broth. Cover and simmer over medium heat about 45 minutes, stirring occasionally, until very tender. Drain any leftover liquid, transfer cooked lentils to a bowl, and stir in chia seeds. Add carrots, potato, onions, arugula, basil, garlic, mustard, oats, breadcrumbs, soy sauce, and salt and pepper, if using. Stir well to make a thick mixture.

2. Place 1 tablespoon of olive oil in a large, cast-iron skillet. Heat well. Form patties by pressing a handful of the lentil mixture into a firm, thin patty. Drop in skillet (four to five per batch), and cook for 7 minutes on medium heat. Turn carefully and cook on the other side for 7 minutes. Repeat process, adding another tablespoon of oil to pan, until all patties are cooked.

3. To make Basil Arugula Cashew Cream, soak the cashews in a covered bowl of water for 3 hours. Drain, and blend with lemon juice and the cup of water until very smooth. Texture should be thick and creamy. Add the arugula and basil, and process until smooth, creamy, and light green in color. Serve Lentil Patties with a dollop of Basil Arugula Cashew Cream. Refrigerate any leftovers in an airtight container for up to three days.

Nutrition for Lentil Patties: 170 calories, 4 g total fat, 1 g saturated fat, 8 g protein, 26 g carbohydrates, 8 g fiber

Nutrition for Basic Arugula Cashew Cream: 100 calories, 8 g total fat, 1 g saturated fat, 3 g protein, 6 g carbohydrates, 1 g fiber

Recipe by Sharon Palmer, RDN | www.sharonpalmer.com

Curried Chickpea Quinoa Loaf

Recipe contributor Sharon Palmer is a plant-based eater and created this modern, plant-based version of a chicken curry and rice dish. This wholesome, flavorful, easy vegetarian/vegan loaf is reminiscent of chana masala. She swapped quinoa for the rice to make it even more interesting. I give it a thumbs up!

MIND foods: Olive oil, vegetables, whole grains, nuts

Yield: 6 servings

Time: 10 minutes to prep; 1 hour to cook; plus 1 hour to chill

Difficulty: Medium

   1 teaspoon extra-virgin olive oil

   1 onion, finely diced

   1 fresh turmeric root or 1 teaspoon dried turmeric, reserving a pinch for sauce

   1½ teaspoons garam masala, divided

   ½ teaspoon plus pinch cumin, divided

   ¼ teaspoon plus pinch red chili flakes, divided

   2 cloves garlic, minced

   1 teaspoon minced ginger

   Pinch sea salt (optional)

   1 cup diced mushrooms

   1 cup chopped fresh greens (e.g., chard, spinach, kale)

   2 tablespoons and 1 teaspoon fresh, chopped parsley

   1½ cups tomato sauce, divided

   2 tablespoons chia seeds

2 cups cooked quinoa

1 cup cooked or canned chickpeas, mashed slightly

⅓ cup chopped cashews

½ cup dry oats

1. Heat oil in a skillet on medium heat and sauté onion for 2 minutes. Add turmeric root, 1 teaspoon garam masala, ½ teaspoon cumin, ¼ teaspoon red chili flakes, garlic, ginger, and salt, if using, and sauté for 1 minute. Add mushrooms, greens, and parsley, and sauté for 2 minutes.

2. Transfer onion mixture to a large bowl. In a separate medium bowl, mix ½ cup tomato sauce with chia seeds and allow to stand for 5 minutes. Meanwhile, add quinoa, chickpeas, cashews, and oats to onion mixture, combine well. Add tomato sauce and chia seeds to the large bowl and mix well, using hands if necessary to distribute ingredients.

3. Spray a loaf pan with nonstick cooking spray and transfer the mixture to the pan, pressing contents into pan firmly. Place in the refrigerator and chill for about 1 hour. Preheat the oven to 350°F and bake for 50 minutes until golden and firm. Allow to cool slightly before slicing it into thick slices.

4. Mix 1 cup tomato sauce with remaining pinch of turmeric, ½ teaspoon of garam masala, pinch of cumin, and pinch of red chili flakes, and heat in a small pot until warmed through. Serve each loaf slice with a ladle of tomato sauce.

Nutrition: 300 calories, 9 g total fat, 1 g saturated fat, 12 g protein, 44 g carbohydrates, 9 g fiber

Recipe by Sharon Palmer, RDN | www.sharonpalmer.com

Red Quinoa and Navy Bean Salad with Toasted Almonds, Cilantro, and Lime Cumin Vinaigrette

Red quinoa is an ancient grain high in both protein and fiber. Paired with navy beans, toasted almonds, yellow zucchini, and a lime cumin vinaigrette, this salad is a healthy and delicious powerhouse.

MIND foods: Whole grains, beans, vegetables, nuts, olive oil

Yield: 8 servings

Time: 10 minutes to prep; 15 minutes to cook

Difficulty: Easy

Salad:

¾ cup water

1 bay leaf

½ cup red quinoa

½ teaspoon kosher salt

1 tablespoon lime juice

1 (15-ounce) can navy beans, drained and rinsed

2 yellow zucchinis, destemmed and cut lengthwise into ½-inch-thick planks

3 tablespoons plus 2 tablespoons extra-virgin olive oil, divided

1 tablespoon minced rosemary

1 teaspoon pimentón (smoked paprika)

¼ cup sliced toasted almonds

¼ cup toasted sunflower seeds

½ cup chopped cilantro

Lime Cumin Vinaigrette:

2 teaspoons minced garlic

1 serrano pepper, seeded and minced

¼ cup lime juice

Zest of 1 lime

3 tablespoons lemon juice

½ teaspoon toasted cumin seed

½ teaspoon kosher salt

¼ teaspoon cayenne pepper

½ cup extra-virgin olive oil

1. For the salad, bring the water and bay leaf to a boil in a small saucepan, and add the quinoa, reduce to a simmer, cover, and cook for 15 minutes. Remove from the heat and let rest for 10 minutes. Fluff with a fork and season with the kosher salt and lime juice. Cool completely and add the beans; set aside.

2. Preheat the grill to high. Place the zucchini in a bowl with 3 tablespoons of the olive oil, rosemary, and pimentón. Toss to combine. Grill on both sides until colored and cooked, about 6 minutes. Remove and cool, and cut into small chunks. Add grilled zucchini to the bowl of beans and quinoa. Add most of the toasted nuts, remaining 2 tablespoons olive oil, and cilantro and toss to combine; set aside some of the toasted nuts for garnish.

3. For the vinaigrette, combine all the ingredients except for the olive oil in a blender and puree until combined. Add the olive oil while the blender is running to create a creamy dressing. Set aside. To finish the salad, pour the vinaigrette over the salad and stir to coat. Serve on a small plate and top with the reserved toasted nuts and a cilantro sprig.

Nutrition: 360 calories, 27 g total fat, 4 g saturated fat, 8 g protein, 24 g carbohydrates, 5 g fiber

Recipe courtesy of The Bean Institute | www.beaninstitute.com

Vegan Shepherd's Pie with Mashed Cauliflower

Hearty and satisfying plant-based comfort food, this dish is so deliciously savory and perfect to enjoy on cold winter's night. It is hearty and healthy, loaded with fiber, plant-based protein, B vitamins, vitamins A and C, and antioxidants. Plus, you'll have leftovers for days as this makes at least eight servings.

MIND foods: Vegetables, olive oil

Yield: 8 servings

Time: 10 minutes to prep; 60 minutes to cook

Difficulty: Medium

> 2 tablespoons extra-virgin olive oil
>
> 1 cup diced onion
>
> 1 cup diced carrot (about 2 carrots)
>
> 1 cup diced parsnip (about 2 parsnips)
>
> ½ teaspoon salt, divided
>
> ½ teaspoon pepper, divided
>
> 2 large cloves garlic, minced
>
> 8 ounces cremini mushrooms, sliced
>
> 4 cups vegetable broth
>
> 1 cup uncooked green lentils, rinsed and drained
>
> 1 bunch sage (about 5 leaves)
>
> 1 bunch thyme (about 3 or 4 sprigs)
>
> 2 tablespoons cornstarch or arrowroot powder
>
> 3 pounds cauliflower florets (about 3 heads cauliflower)
>
> ⅓ cup almond milk
>
> 3 tablespoons vegan buttery spread

1. In a Dutch oven, heat olive oil over medium heat. Add onion, carrot, and parsnip and cook for 7 to 10 minutes, or until onions

are translucent and veggies are slightly tender. Add ¼ teaspoon of salt and ¼ teaspoon of pepper. Stir in garlic and mushrooms and cook for another 5 minutes (stirring occasionally), or until mushrooms are tender and lightly browned. Add vegetable broth, lentils, sage, and thyme, and reduce heat and let simmer for 35 to 45 minutes, or until lentils are tender.

2. To thicken the lentil mixture, add cornstarch or arrowroot to a heaping spoonful of the lentil mixture in a separate bowl. Whisk together. Add thickened mixture back to the pot and whisk in. Add salt and pepper to taste.

3. Preheat the oven to 425°F. Meanwhile, steam cauliflower florets until fork tender and transfer to a food processor (you may need to do this in batches depending on size of food processor). Add almond milk and vegan buttery spread, and pulse to a smooth and creamy puree. Add remaining ¼ teaspoon each of salt and pepper, plus more to taste. Transfer lentil mixture to a 9 x 13-inch baking dish or a 2-quart baking dish. Carefully spread mashed cauliflower evenly over top. Bake at 425°F for 10 minutes and then transfer to the broiler for 5 minutes, or until cauliflower is crisp and starting to turn golden brown. Remove from oven and let cool briefly before serving.

Nutrition: 250 calories, 9 g total fat, 1 g saturated fat, 13 g protein, 35 g carbohydrates, 12 g fiber

Recipe by Kara Lydon, RD, LDN, RYT | www.karalydon.com

Tzatziki-Smothered Sweet Potatoes

This baked sweet potato topped with tangy, garlicky tzatziki, crunchy garbanzo beans, fresh tomato, diced onion, and chopped parsley is the perfect alternative to a traditional cheesy baked potato. Bursting with flavor and nutritious ingredients, this is a baked potato you can feel good about.

MIND foods: Vegetables, beans, olive oil

Yield: 4 servings

Time: 45 minutes

Difficulty: Medium

Greek Island Tzatziki Sauce:

1½ cups plain Greek yogurt

4 garlic cloves

½ peeled, deseeded, and diced cucumber, divided

2 tablespoons lemon juice

2 tablespoons extra-virgin olive oil

1 tablespoon white wine vinegar

½ teaspoon sea salt

¼ teaspoon pepper

¼ teaspoon fresh dill

Crunchy Oregano Garbanzo Beans:

1 (15-ounce) can garbanzo beans, drained, rinsed, and dried

1 teaspoon olive oil

1 teaspoon dried oregano

¼ teaspoon red pepper flakes

½ teaspoon garlic powder

¾ teaspoon onion powder

½ teaspoon ground cumin

½ teaspoon sea salt

Basic Baked Sweet Potatoes:

4 sweet potatoes, cut in half lengthwise

1–2 tablespoons extra-virgin olive oil

1 large tomato, chopped

½ red onion, thinly sliced

¼ cup parsley, chopped

1. Make the tzatziki sauce. (This can be done ahead, and the flavors develop better over time.) In a food processor, combine the Greek yogurt, garlic, half of the diced cucumber, lemon juice, olive oil, white wine vinegar, sea salt, pepper, and dill. Process until smooth. In a large bowl, fold the remaining diced cucumber into the smooth tzatziki sauce. Top with additional drizzle of olive oil and pepper, if desired. Refrigerate until ready for use.

2. Preheat the oven to 400°F. Prep Crunchy Oregano Garbanzo Beans. In a large bowl, combine the garbanzo beans, olive oil, dried oregano, red pepper flakes, garlic powder, onion powder, cumin, and sea salt. Mix until well coated. Spread beans on a large baking sheet lined with parchment paper.

3. Next, prep the Basic Baked Sweet Potatoes. Massage sweet potatoes halves with olive oil. On a baking sheet lined with foil, place sweet potatoes flesh side down. Place baking sheets for garbanzo beans and sweet potatoes into the preheated oven and bake for 15 minutes. Shake garbanzo bean pan to turn the beans, and bake for another 10 minutes until crisp. Flip sweet potatoes, and bake for another 15 minutes until fork tender. Top sweet potatoes with tzatziki, garbanzo beans, tomato, red onion, and parsley. Serve.

Nutrition: 400 calories, 14 g total fat, 2 g saturated fat, 15 g protein, 54 g carbohydrates, 11 g fiber

Recipe by Amari Thomsen, MS, RD, LDN | www.eatchicchicago.com

Roasted Chicken with Fennel, Carrots, and Dried Plums

Juicy, savory, and flavorful roasted chicken with fennel, carrots, onions, and dried plums is a one-pan meal that's full of flavor thanks to various herbs and spices. Easy enough for a weeknight meal and elegant enough for company.

MIND foods: Vegetables, poultry, olive oil

Yield: 8 to 10

Time: 10 minutes to prep; 1 hour to 1 hour 15 minutes to cook

Difficulty: Easy

1 pound carrots, peeled, halved lengthwise, and cut into ½-inch chunks (about 3 cups)

1 large fennel bulb, sliced (about 3 cups)

2 onions, sliced into half moons

3 tablespoons extra-virgin olive oil, divided

1 tablespoon chopped fresh rosemary (or 1 teaspoon dried)

1 teaspoon dried marjoram

1 teaspoon chili powder

2 whole bone-in chicken breasts (or 4 split bone-in chicken breasts)

1 tablespoon lemon juice

2 cloves garlic, chopped

¾ cup dry white wine or low-sodium chicken broth, divided

Kosher salt and pepper, to taste

1 cup dried plums (prunes), chopped

1. Preheat the oven to 400°F. Spread carrots, fennel, and onions on the bottom of a large roasting pan. Toss with 1 tablespoon of the olive oil.

2. In a small bowl, whisk remaining 2 tablespoons of olive oil with the rosemary, marjoram, and chili powder to form a paste. Spread on chicken breasts, being sure to get under the skin.

Place on a roasting rack over the vegetables. Drizzle lemon juice over chicken breasts and sprinkle with chopped garlic. Pour ½ cup of wine or broth around chicken (not on top). Sprinkle chicken and vegetables with salt and pepper. Roast chicken and vegetables for 35 minutes.

3. Baste top of chicken, toss in prunes, and cook another 15 to 20 minutes until chicken skin is nicely browned and internal temperature is 150°F. Let chicken rest. (Note: Food safety recommendations for chicken is an internal temp of 165°F; however, chicken continues cooking after removed from the oven, so to retain moisture, remove it at 150°F.) If vegetables need to cook longer, transfer chicken to a cutting board to rest, and continue roasting vegetables for another 5 to 10 minutes. Pour pan drippings into saucepan. Add remaining ¼ cup wine or broth. Simmer for 5 to 10 minutes until gravy reduces. To serve, slice chicken off bone and serve with vegetable/dried plum mixture with gravy on top.

Nutrition: 420 calories, 12 g total fat, 2.5 g saturated fat, 54 g protein, 19 g carbohydrates, 3 g fiber

Recipe by Jessica Fishman Levinson, MS, RDN, CDN | www.nutritioulicious.com

Roasted Potatoes, String Beans, and Shredded Chicken Salad

This salad offers a tasty marriage of nutrients with a comforting starch from potatoes (optional: swap in sweet potatoes), lean protein from the shredded chicken breast, and a splash of colorful goodness from the string beans. It's simple to assemble and you can save the leftovers for another meal.

MIND foods: Poultry, vegetables, olive oil

Yield: 4 servings

Time: 25 minutes to prep; 45 minutes to cook

Difficulty: Easy

2 (6-ounce) boneless, skinless chicken breasts

1 pound red potatoes, washed and quartered

1 tablespoon extra-virgin olive oil

2 large garlic cloves, diced

1 teaspoon salt

Dash pepper

2 sprigs fresh rosemary, coarsely chopped

2 cups string beans, rinsed and trimmed

For dressing:

1 tablespoon extra-virgin olive oil

1 tablespoon balsamic vinegar

1 teaspoon Dijon mustard

1 teaspoon smoked paprika

1. Preheat the oven to 400°F. Place chicken breasts on a cookie sheet in the oven. Roast for about 30 minutes (depends on thickness), checking with a meat thermometer that it reaches 165°F. Remove from oven and let cool a bit before shredding.

2. Toss potatoes with olive oil, garlic, salt, pepper, and rosemary in an oven-safe baking dish or roasting pan and cook for 20 minutes in the oven. Add the string beans, toss with potatoes, and return to oven to cook for another 20 minutes. Check for doneness; potatoes should be tender and brown, string beans should be slightly wilted. Remove from oven and allow to cool 5 minutes. Whisk together the dressing ingredients. To plate dishes, divide potatoes and green beans on each plate, and top with 3 ounces of shredded chicken. Drizzle with dressing and serve.

Nutrition: 270 calories, 8 g total fat, 1 g saturated fat, 16 g protein, 36 g carbohydrates, 5 g fiber

Recipe by Vicki Shanta Retelny, RDN, LDN | www.simplecravingsrealfood.com

Turkey-Ginger Sliders

Bursting with flavor, this versatile recipe can be used to make healthier burgers, meatballs, or appetizers. The patties freeze well for easy make-ahead weeknight meals.

MIND foods: Poultry, vegetables, whole grains, olive oil

Yield: 6 sliders

Time: 10 minutes to prep; 20 minutes to cook

Difficulty: Easy

> *10-ounce 95% lean ground turkey*
>
> *1 (1-inch) piece ginger, minced*
>
> *1 shallot, minced*
>
> *1 tablespoon tomato paste*
>
> *Salt and pepper, to taste*
>
> *2 teaspoons extra-virgin olive oil*
>
> *1 medium cucumber, sliced on the diagonal*
>
> *6 whole grain slider buns*

1. In a medium bowl, combine ground turkey, ginger, shallot, and tomato paste. Season with salt and pepper. Wearing plastic gloves, mix together until just combined. Form six patties, about ¼-inch thick.

2. Heat olive oil in medium pan on medium-high heat until hot. Add patties and cook for 1 to 2 minutes per side or until cooked through. Transfer to a paper-towel-lined plate to drain. This recipe makes enough for three people to have two sliders each. Assemble sliders by placing cucumber slices and patties between buns.

Nutrition: 350 calories, 14 g total fat, 3 g saturated fat, 25 g protein, 33 g carbohydrates, 5 g fiber

Roasted Halibut with Spicy Black Bean Cakes

In this Latin-influenced dish, the silky richness of halibut is offset by the vibrantly flavorful black bean cakes. The spiciness of the jalapeños plays nicely with the richness of the sweet potato in these bean cakes to make this a great side for the halibut. A squeeze of lime at the end brings it all together.

MIND foods: Olive oil, vegetables, beans, fish

Yield: 8 servings

Time: 40 minutes to prep; 20 minutes to cook; plus 50 minutes to chill

Difficulty: Medium

Bean cakes:

   4 tablespoons extra-virgin olive oil, divided

   1 white onion, peeled and diced

   2 tablespoons garlic cloves, crushed and chopped

   ¼ cup jalapeño peppers, stemmed and minced

   2 teaspoons toasted ground cumin

   3 cups cooked black beans, divided

   1 teaspoon kosher salt

   1 teaspoon ground pepper

   2 cups sweet potato, peeled and grated

   2 eggs, lightly beaten

   ¾ cup whole grain toasted breadcrumbs, plus extra for coating finished cakes

Halibut:

   2 pounds halibut fillet, skinned and portioned into 4-ounce pieces

   Salt and pepper, to taste

   1 tablespoon toasted ground fennel seed

   ¼ cup extra-virgin olive oil

   1 lime, quartered, to serve

1. For the bean cakes, heat 2 tablespoons of olive oil in a small skillet over medium heat. Cook onion until softened, about 1 minute. Stir in garlic, jalapeños, and toasted cumin; cook until fragrant, about 2 minutes. Transfer contents of skillet to a large bowl. Stir in 2 cups of cooked black beans and mash with a fork. Season with salt and pepper. Add sweet potatoes, eggs, remaining 1 cup of the cooked black beans, and breadcrumbs. Mix again carefully just to combine and chill for 30 minutes.

2. Divide into 16 small balls and flatten into square patties. Lightly grease baking sheet with 2 tablespoons of olive oil. Dip patties into breadcrumbs to coat and place on oiled sheet pan; chill for 20 minutes. Preheat the oven to 450°F. Place bean cakes in the oven and roast for 10 minutes, or until the cakes start to lightly brown.

3. Meanwhile, pat the halibut fillets dry with paper towels. Season the halibut portions generously with salt, pepper, and the toasted fennel seed. Heat ¼ cup of olive oil over medium-high heat in a large oven-proof pan until hot but not smoking. Slip the halibut pieces into the pan and cook until the bottom side is golden and the edges of the fish start to look opaque, about 3 minutes. Flip the fish fillets over and place in the oven for 2 to 3 minutes, or until the fillets are just opaque in the center. Serve the fish with warm roasted black bean cakes and fresh lime wedges.

Nutrition: 430 calories, 17 g total fat, 3 g saturated fat, 31 g protein, 38 g carbohydrates, 9 g fiber

Recipe courtesy of The Bean Institute | www.beaninstitute.com

Almond-Crusted Baked Salmon

Salmon is one of the richest sources of omega-3. A family favorite, this simple, delicious salmon dish goes well with wild rice and roasted asparagus, but choose the whole grain and vegetable side of your choice. Enjoy.

MIND foods: Fish, nuts

Yield: 4 servings

Time: 10 minutes to prep; 10 minutes to cook

Difficulty: Easy

> 2 tablespoons Dijon mustard
>
> Zest of 1 lemon
>
> 1 tablespoon chopped herbs of choice (dill, lemon thyme, chives, parsley)
>
> 4 (6-ounce) thick-cut salmon fillets
>
> Pepper
>
> ¼ cup chopped almonds

1. Preheat the oven to 400°F. Mix the mustard, zest, and herbs together on a plate. Pepper the salmon, dip in the mustard-zest-herb mixture, then roll in the crushed almonds. Spray a baking pan with cooking spray, add salmon, and place in oven for 10 minutes. Cover and let rest for 5 minutes.

Nutrition: 290 calories, 17 g total fat, 2 g saturated fat, 29 g protein, 4 g carbohydrates, 2 g fiber

Recipe by Madeline Basler, MS, RDN, CDN | www.realyounutrition.com

Grilled Apricot-Glazed Salmon

This delicious and nutritious salmon recipe provides an abundance of healthy omega-3 fatty acids for brain and heart health and requires hardly any cleanup. Salmon goes well with almost any grain, and this rich-tasting fish tastes great with a hearty grain like brown rice. Serve this dish over a bed of greens, hot or at room temperature.

MIND foods: Fish, olive oil

Yield: 4 servings

Time: 10 minutes to prep; 10 to 15 minutes to cook

Difficulty: Easy

> 1⅓ pounds salmon fillets (choose wild salmon when available)
>
> ¼ teaspoon pepper
>
> 1 tablespoon extra-virgin olive oil
>
> 1 clove garlic, minced
>
> ⅓ cup 100% fruit apricot spread
>
> 1 tablespoon Dijon mustard
>
> ½ cup low-sodium vegetable broth

1. Preheat the grill to medium heat (if unable to grill, see alternative option to bake in the oven below). Pat salmon dry with a paper towel and cut into four equal servings. Season the skinless side of salmon with pepper. Place each piece of salmon on a double layer of foil with skin side down. Fold the sides of the foil up so that the cooking liquid will not run out.

2. In a small bowl, whisk together the rest of the ingredients. Pour the liquid over the four pieces of salmon so that the glaze is distributed equally. Seal each foil by folding as if you were wrapping a gift. Slide the foil packets onto the grill and close the lid. Cook until the salmon is cooked through, about 10 minutes. Let it rest for 2 minutes and then unwrap and serve.

Alternative cooking method:

1. Preheat the oven to 400°F. Line a shallow baking pan with aluminum foil. Place salmon skin-side down on foil and follow the remainder of the recipe, except leave the foil open. Bake for 15 minutes or until salmon flakes easily with a fork.

Nutrition: 300 calories, 12 g total fat, 2 g saturated fat, 33 g protein, 14 g carbohydrates, 1 g fiber

Recipe by Layne Lieberman, MS, RDN, CDN | www.worldrd.com

Mustard-Dill Crusted Salmon

With only three ingredients, this is such a simple recipe that still manages to impress.

MIND foods: Fish

Yield: 4 servings

Time: 10 minutes of prep; 18 to 22 minutes to cook

Difficulty: Easy

> 4 (4- to 6-ounce) salmon fillets
>
> 1 bunch fresh dill, washed and patted dry
>
> 1 cup whole grain mustard

1. Preheat the oven to 425°F. Pat salmon dry with paper towels and place on baking sheet. Tear off top half of dill (discard stems), and place a large handful in a blender or food processor. Add mustard and blend until dill is chopped. Spread 1 to 2 tablespoons mustard-dill sauce on each salmon fillet. Place baking sheet in oven, on a center shelf. Bake for 18 to 22 minutes, or until fish is just cooked through and flaky.

Nutrition: 350 calories, 17 g total fat, 3 g saturated fat, 32 g protein, 14 g carbohydrates, 1 g fiber

Recipe by Chef Allison Schaaff, MS, RD, LD | www.prepdish.com

Raspberry, Sriracha, and Ginger Glazed Salmon

Kick your heart-healthy salmon up a notch with fantastic Raspberry Sriracha Ginger Glaze.

MIND foods: Fish, olive oil, berries

Yield: 4 servings

Time: 10 minutes to prep; 20 minutes to cook

Difficulty: Medium

Salmon:

4 (5-ounce) salmon fillets

2 teaspoons extra-virgin olive oil

1 teaspoon kosher salt

Pepper, to taste

Raspberry Sriracha Ginger Glaze:

4 ounces or about 1 cup ginger, peeled and sliced ¼-inch thick

4 cups frozen raspberries, thawed

1 cup mirin

1 cup apple juice

1 cup water

1–2 teaspoons (adjust heat to desired level) sriracha sauce

1. Preheat the oven to 400°F. Season salmon with olive oil, salt, and pepper. Set aside.

2. Make the Raspberry Sriracha Ginger Glaze. Combine all ingredients in a medium saucepan and cook over medium-high heat. Bring to a boil, reduce heat, and simmer until liquid is reduced by one-third and slightly thickened. (Note: the sriracha sauce increases in heat level when the sauce is reduced.) Remove from heat and strain through a fine-mesh strainer into two small-sized bowls. (Note: This can be made in advance and refrigerated until needed.)

3. Brush the first batch of Raspberry Sriracha Ginger Glaze onto seasoned salmon portions prior to baking. Place salmon filets on a baking sheet and transfer to a hot oven. Bake for about 8 to 12 minutes until salmon is done. Remove sheet from oven. At the end of the baking, prior to serving, brush the second batch of glaze onto the salmon. Use about ½ to 1 ounce of glaze per salmon portion.

Glazed Salmon (includes 1 ounce of glaze) Nutrition: 310 calories, 13 g total fat, 2 g saturated fat, 33 g protein, 14 g carbohydrates, 1 g fiber

Raspberry Sriracha Ginger Glaze Nutrition (1 oz): 60 calories, 0 g total fat, 0 g saturated fat, 1 g protein, 14 g carbohydrates, 1 g fiber

Recipe courtesy of National Processed Raspberry Council | www.redrazz.org

Pistachio-Crusted Trout

This is an easy recipe to get more seafood on the table using simple ingredients with a lot of flavor. The mild flavor of trout makes it a crowd-pleaser.

MIND foods: Fish, nuts

Yield: 4 servings

Time: 10 minutes to prep; 20 minutes to cook

Difficulty: Easy

> 4 (6–8 ounce) trout fillets
>
> 1 fresh lemon
>
> Pinch salt
>
> Pepper, to taste
>
> 1 cup shelled pistachios, crushed

1. Preheat the oven to 350°F. Pat fillets dry with paper towels. Place skin side down on an oiled baking sheet. Squeeze the juice of the lemon onto the skinless side. Sprinkle with salt and pepper. Add the pistachios to a blender or food processor and pulse five to seven times until they make a course, breadcrumb-like texture. If you don't want to dirty your blender, you can also place nuts in a plastic sandwich bag and crush them with the bottom of a cup or rolling pin. Rub the pistachios onto the exposed side of the fish and transfer the pan to the oven. Bake for 20 to 25 minutes or until fish flakes easily with a fork.

Optional: Transfer the fish to the broiler for the last couple of minutes of cooking to brown the pistachios.

Nutrition: 280 calories, 18 g total fat, 2.5 g saturated fat, 23 g protein, 9 g carbohydrates, 3 g fiber

Recipe by Meri Raffetto, RDN | www.reallivingnutrition.com

Tango Fish Tacos

This recipe is not only easy to make, but healthy because it is made with fish and the freshest ingredients for the salsa. It can also have as little or big a kick as you want by varying the level of spices used.

MIND foods: Fish, olive oil, whole grains, vegetables

Yield: 6 servings

Time: 15 minutes to prep; 15 minutes to cook

Difficulty: Medium

1 pound cod or haddock

¼ cup extra-virgin olive oil

½ teaspoon chili powder

½ teaspoon paprika

½ teaspoon cayenne pepper

2 teaspoons dried oregano

Salt and pepper, to taste

8 (6-inch) corn tortillas

Salsa:

1 mango, diced

1 jalapeño pepper, chopped fine

½ medium red onion, chopped

3 Roma tomatoes, chopped

1 cup chopped cilantro

½ teaspoon salt

1–2 tablespoons lime juice, to taste

1 teaspoon lime zest

1. Preheat oven to 400°F. Combine the salsa ingredients in a medium bowl. Set aside.

2. In a small bowl, combine fish seasonings. Brush the fish with olive oil and sprinkle spice mixture generously over fillets. Place on a baking sheet, and bake for 8 to 9 minutes or until the fish flakes off with a fork. Remove fish from the oven and let rest for 2 to 3 minutes. Warm tortillas for 1 to 2 minutes in the oven before removing. Cut fish into strips. Top each tortilla with fish and salsa.

Nutrition: 390 calories, 22 g total fat, 1 g saturated fat, 15 g protein, 29 g carbohydrates, 13 g fiber

Recipe by Kim Melton, RDN | www.nutritionproconsulting.com

Sriracha Shrimp with Zoodles

This spicy shrimp dish is made with minimal ingredients and is ready in under 30 minutes. It's a low-calorie, protein-rich meal. Sriracha is a type of hot sauce originating in Thailand that is made primarily of chili pepper paste, distilled vinegar, and garlic. It has an intense flavor and spicy-hot heat that many people have grown to love and even crave. However, if you're new to sriracha, start slowly and with small amounts.

MIND foods: Vegetables, olive oil, fish

Yield: 2 servings

Time: 8 minutes to prep; 12 minutes to cook

Difficulty: Easy

1 small zucchini

1 small yellow/summer squash

1 teaspoon olive oil

½ sweet onion, thinly sliced

1 teaspoon fresh garlic, minced

1 teaspoon fresh ginger, grated

1 dozen raw shrimp, peeled

1–2 teaspoons sriracha sauce

1. Slice zucchini and yellow squash in a spiralizer, making noodles, or, if you will, zoodles (see alternate method below). Cut spiraled vegetable noodles into 4 to 6-inch pieces. In a large skillet or wok, heat olive oil over medium heat. Add onion, garlic, and ginger to oil and cook for about 3 minutes until onion softens. Add in shrimp, and cook until pink and opaque, about 5 minutes. Add in spiralized zucchini and yellow squash to skillet, and cook for about 3 minutes to soften. Add in sriracha sauce and stir to coat.

Alternate method for making zoodles:

1. What's a zoodle you ask? Zoodles are made from zucchini that has been cut into strips resembling spaghetti. A spiralizer is often used to create these vegetable "noodles." There are many types of spiralizers. Some are simple handheld gadgets that resemble a large pencil sharpener, while other spiralizers sit on your kitchen counter. If you don't own one of these spiralizers you can either shave the vegetables into ribbons with a vegetable peeler, or use a julienne peeler, mandolin, or knife to create your noodles.

Nutrition: 190 calories, 7 g total fat, 1 g saturated fat, 19 g protein, 16 g carbohydrates, 5 g fiber

Recipe by Jennifer Lynn-Pullman MA, RDN, LDN | www.nourishedsimply.com

Grilled Shrimp Skewers with Rosemary White Beans and Sautéed Swiss Chard

The white beans in this dish really take on the flavors of the chili and fresh herbs. The rosemary brings beautiful aromatics to this versatile dish that can be easily scaled to an entrée or appetizer portion. Grilling the shrimp on the rosemary skewers continues the flavor profile throughout the dish and creates an elegant presentation option.

MIND foods: Beans, olive oil, fish, leafy greens

Yield: 8 servings

Time: 2 hours, 10 minutes, plus overnight soaking time

Difficulty: Medium

Beans:

> 1 pound dried white cannellini beans
>
> ⅓ cup extra-virgin olive oil
>
> 1 fresh (6-inch) branch rosemary
>
> 2 bay leaves
>
> ½ teaspoon red pepper flakes
>
> Pepper, to taste
>
> 1 teaspoon kosher salt

Shrimp:

> 24 large shrimp (about 1 pound), shelled and deveined
>
> ¼ cup extra-virgin olive oil
>
> 1 tablespoon thyme, minced
>
> 8 rosemary skewers
>
> Sea salt, to taste

Swiss chard:

> 3 tablespoons extra-virgin olive oil
>
> 6 tablespoons shallots, minced
>
> 2 tablespoons garlic, minced

2 bunches white, red, or rainbow Swiss chard, stemmed and torn into pieces

1 teaspoon salt

½ teaspoon pepper

2 fluid ounces white wine

1. Sort and wash the beans of any debris and dust, then refrigerate them overnight soaked in three times the volume of water as beans. Discard any beans that float or appear wrinkled and misshapen. Drain the soaking water and reserve. Place the beans in a 3-quart pot with just enough soaking water to cover the beans. Bring the beans to a boil and skim the pot well of any foam that rises. Reduce the heat to the barest simmer, add the remaining ingredients except for the salt, and cover the pot with a tight-fitting lid. It is possible, with a low fire, that the beans will take 2 to 2½ hours to cook. Check the water level on the beans every 20 minutes and add more hot water as needed to keep them covered. As the beans approach tenderness, give them ever less liquid—the ideal would be a finished pot of moist, tender beans without excessive cooking liquid. Once the beans are tender, add the salt and adjust the seasoning. Set aside in a warm place until the rest of the dish is prepared. If you intend to store the beans for later, keep them in their cooking liquid, covered, and refrigerate for up to four days.

2. While beans are simmering, in a medium bowl, combine shrimp, oil, and thyme. Cover and refrigerate for 2 to 6 hours. For rosemary skewers, pull half of the leaves off each stalk so that leaves remain on one end. Sharpen the other end into a point with a paring knife. Thread three shrimp onto the pointed end of each skewer.

3. For the chard, heat the olive oil in a large sauté pan over medium-high heat. Add the shallots and garlic to the pan and

sweat until translucent, about 5 minutes. Add the chard to the pan, and season with salt and pepper. Sauté until just barely wilted, about 5 to 7 minutes. Sauté in batches if necessary. Add the white wine to the pan and cover. Steam the chard until the spines are tender and the liquid has almost evaporated, about 5 minutes.

4. To cook the shrimp, heat a grill, grill pan, or broiler. Cook shrimp about 3 minutes per side, until they turn opaque and start to curl slightly.

5. To serve, place a small amount of the Swiss chard in the middle of a plate and top with some of the cooked beans. Place a cooked shrimp skewer on top and season with the sea salt.

Nutrition: 440 calories, 22 g total fat, 3 g saturated fat, 22 g protein, 38 g carbohydrates, 10 g fiber

Recipe courtesy of The Bean Institute | www.beaninstitute.com

Salads & Soups

Strawberry and Baby Arugula Salad

This simple salad lets the quality of the ingredients really shine through, so be sure to choose ripe, red strawberries and fresh baby arugula leaves. It's so quick and easy to put together as a side salad, or could be converted to a main dish with salmon or chicken on top.

MIND foods: Leafy greens, berries, olive oil

Yield: 4 servings

Time: 10 minutes

Difficulty: Easy

    4 cups prewashed baby arugula

    2 cups sliced strawberries

Dressing:

    1 tablespoon champagne vinegar

    ¼ cup extra-virgin olive oil

    ½ lemon, juiced

    Salt and pepper, to taste

1. In a medium bowl, combine champagne vinegar, olive oil, lemon juice, and salt and pepper, and whisk until well combined. In a large bowl, add arugula. Pour dressing over greens and massage gently with clean hands for 1 minute. Add the strawberries

into the large salad bowl and gently fold them into the salad.
This salad also works great with baby kale in place of the baby
arugula.

Nutrition: 150 calories, 14 g total fat, 2 g saturated fat, 1 g protein, 8 g
carbohydrates, 2 g fiber

Kale Apple Carrot Salad

*This salad is super simple to make and kid-friendly. It is a tasty way to help
your family enjoy raw veggies and receive the benefits of apple cider vinegar.*

MIND foods: Leafy greens, vegetables, olive oil

Yield: 6 servings

Time: 11 minutes

Difficulty: Easy

> *2 cups raw kale, cut into fine ribbons*
>
> *2 honey crisp apples, julienned (can substitute any sweet apple)*
>
> *2 heaping cups julienned carrots*
>
> *3 tablespoons apple cider vinegar*
>
> *2 tablespoons extra-virgin olive oil*
>
> *1 tablespoon honey*
>
> *¼ teaspoon sea salt*
>
> *Pinch of pepper*

1. In a mixing bowl, toss kale, apples, and carrots together. Set
   aside. In a small jar, pour vinegar, oil, honey, salt, and pepper.
   Seal lid on the jar and shake vigorously to combine. Pour
   dressing on top of salad and either gently toss or massage into
   mixture with hands. Serve immediately.

Nutrition: 90 calories, 5 g total fat, 1 g saturated fat, 1 g protein, 13 g
carbohydrates, 3 g fiber

Recipe by Jenna Braddock, MSH, RDN, CSSD, LD/N |
www.JennaBraddock.com

Golden Kale Tahini Salad

This salad combines silky kale greens with creamy tahini dressing and sweet golden raisins. Spicy roasted garbanzo beans provide an added crunch and serve as a fun alternative to croutons.

MIND foods: Leafy greens, olive oil, vegetables, beans

Yield: 5 servings

Time: 10 minutes to prep; 30 minutes to cook

Difficulty: Easy

Roasted garbanzo beans:

1 (15-ounce) can garbanzo beans, rinsed and drained

1 tablespoon extra-virgin olive oil

½ teaspoon ground cumin

⅛ teaspoon cayenne pepper

Pinch sea salt

Salad:

5 cups chopped kale

1 tablespoon extra-virgin olive oil

Pinch sea salt

1 cup golden raisins

1 Persian cucumber, sliced

2 avocados, diced

Lemon Tahini Dressing (can be made ahead of time):

1 lemon, juiced

3 tablespoons water

3 tablespoons tahini

⅛ teaspoon cayenne pepper

1. Preheat the oven to 400°F.

2. Prep the garbanzo beans. In a medium bowl, combine the garbanzo beans, olive oil, cumin, cayenne pepper, and sea salt.

Spread the garbanzo beans in an even layer on a rimmed baking sheet and bake in the oven for 30 minutes, stirring once halfway through baking.

3. While the garbanzo beans are roasting, place the kale in a large bowl with the olive oil and sea salt. Gently massage the kale with your hands to tenderize the leaves (it helps to soften the bitter flavor).

4. Next, prepare the dressing. In a small bowl, whisk together the lemon juice, water, tahini, and cayenne pepper. Set aside. Once the garbanzo beans have finished roasting, add the raisins, cucumber, avocados, and garbanzo beans to the kale. Top the salad with the dressing and toss.

Nutrition: 320 calories, 18 g total fat, 2.5 g saturated fat, 9 g protein, 41 g carbohydrates, 10 g fiber

Recipe by McKenzie Hall Jones, RDN | www.nourishRDs.com

Broccoli Slaw Salad with Flaxseeds and Hemp Seeds

This salad offers a healthier spin on coleslaw, combining flavonoid-rich broccoli and lycopene-packed tomato with avocado, offering healthy monounsaturated fats. The almonds, seeds, and oil also provide healthy fats. The salad makes a great side dish; or for a complete meal, top it with grilled salmon or tofu and pair with a side of brown rice or quinoa.

MIND foods: Vegetables, olive oil, nuts

Yield: 4 servings

Time: 5 minutes

Difficulty: Easy

> 12 ounces broccoli slaw mix
> 1 avocado, diced

1 plum tomato, diced

1 tablespoon rice vinegar

1 tablespoon plus 1 teaspoon extra-virgin olive oil

1 teaspoon honey

2 tablespoons slivered almonds

1½ tablespoons flaxseeds

1½ tablespoons hemp seeds

Salt and pepper, to taste

1. In a large bowl, combine broccoli slaw with avocado and tomato. In a small bowl, mix vinegar, oil, and honey. Toss with broccoli slaw mixture. Top with almonds and seeds, and sprinkle with pepper and salt.

Nutrition: 210 calories, 16 g total fat, 2 g saturated fat, 6 g protein, 14 g carbohydrates, 7 g fiber

Recipe by Amy Gorin, MS, RDN | www.amydgorin.com

Fattoush Salad

Fattoush is a bread salad that is usually made with toasted or fried pieces of pita bread, combined with mixed greens and other vegetables. Not to worry, you won't find any fried foods in this recipe. An easy Middle Eastern chopped salad with loads of vegetables, a homemade lemon vinaigrette, and toasted whole grain flatbread, this fattoush salad recipe is a must-try.

MIND foods: Whole grains, olive oil, leafy greens, vegetables

Yield: 2 servings

Time: 10 minutes

Difficulty: Easy

Salad:

1 whole wheat pita

2 teaspoons extra-virgin olive oil

½ teaspoon garlic powder

1 head of romaine lettuce, chopped

1 medium tomato, chopped

½ cucumber, chopped

½ orange bell pepper, cut into strips

½ cup parsley, finely chopped

¼ cup green onion, diced

Dressing:

¼ cup lemon juice

2 tablespoons extra-virgin olive oil

2 cloves garlic, minced

1 teaspoon sumac

1. Preheat oven to 400°F. Brush pita with olive oil and sprinkle with garlic powder. Bake pita in oven until crisp. Take out and break into bite-size pieces. Mix together all vegetables for salad. Whisk together all ingredients for dressing. When ready to serve, toss together the flatbread chips with the salad and dressing.

Nutrition: 300 calories, 18 g total fat, 2.5 g saturated fat, 7 g protein, 35 g carbohydrates, 7 g fiber

Recipe by Amanda Hernandez, MA, RD | www.nutritionistreviews.com

Lacinato Kale and Red Grapefruit Salad

The deep flavors of dark leafy greens and the brightness of citrus come into season just in time to bring cheer to gray days. This salad pops with so many flavors. Kale will provide tons of antioxidant vitamin A, and the citrus in the dressing and the grapefruit take care of vitamin C. The hazelnuts are a delicious source of unsaturated fats to help absorb fat-soluble vitamin A, as well as some protein and B vitamins.

MIND foods: Nuts, leafy greens, vegetables, olive oil

Yield: 4 servings

Time: 8 minutes to prep; 12 minutes to cook

Difficulty: Easy

> *4 ounces hazelnuts (aka filberts)*
>
> *1 bunch lacinato kale, torn into bite-size pieces*
>
> *1 stalk fennel, cut into ¼-inch slices*
>
> *2 tablespoons chopped dill (optional)*
>
> *1 red grapefruit*

Dressing:

> *¼ cup extra-virgin olive oil*
>
> *1 tablespoon pinot noir red wine vinegar*
>
> *1 tablespoon honey*
>
> *1 lemon, juiced*
>
> *1 lime, juiced*
>
> *Salt and pepper, to taste*

1. Preheat oven to 350°F. Evenly spread hazelnuts on rimmed baking sheet. Roast hazelnuts for 10 minutes, stirring halfway through.

2. Meanwhile, in a large bowl, combine the kale, fennel, and dill (if using). Set aside.

3. Prepare the dressing. Whisk all dressing ingredients until combined. Add dressing to the large bowl and gently massage salad for 1 to 2 minutes (it softens the kale's bitterness). Cut away the peel and pith of the grapefruit, and remove the fleshy segments so that there is no skin or pith. Fold grapefruit segments into main salad (it's OK if some of them are broken in halves or even thirds). Top with toasted hazelnuts.

Nutrition: 290 calories, 23 g total fat, 3 g saturated fat, 6 g protein, 21 g carbohydrates, 4 g fiber

Baby Greens Salad with Banana-Curry Vinaigrette

A bed of baby greens tossed with ribboned carrots, diced bananas, slivers of red onion, English cucumbers, and toasted pistachios, in a creamy, dairy-free Banana-Curry Vinaigrette is a surprising treat for the palate. People don't always think of fruit in green salads, but they add a naturally sweet dimension to balance more acidic and earthy flavors. The natural sweetness of bananas in this salad means there's absolutely no need for any added sugar from dressings, and the fiber in bananas and all those veggies offer a prebiotic paradise for gut health. Last but not least, there are several different textures going on in this salad to keep things interesting.

MIND foods: Nuts, leafy greens, vegetables, olive oil

Yield: 4 servings

Time: 10 minutes to prep; 5 minutes to combine

Difficulty: Easy

Salad:

    ¼ cup shelled pistachios

    4 cups organic baby greens

    ½ cup diced English cucumbers

    1 medium carrot, peeled into ribbons

    ½ small red onion, thinly sliced

    1 large just-ripe banana, diced

Banana Curry Vinaigrette Dressing:

    1 tablespoon curry powder

    ¼ cup extra-virgin olive oil

    2 tablespoons champagne vinegar

    ½ small ripe banana

    Salt and pepper, to taste

    Remaining ½ banana, sliced, as garnish (optional)

1. To make the dressing, toast curry powder in a small pan over medium heat until fragrant, 1 to 2 minutes. Remove from heat and transfer to a medium bowl. Wipe pan clean.

2. To the medium bowl, add olive oil and vinegar and whisk to combine. Puree ½ small banana until completely smooth, and slowly add to curry-oil-vinegar mixture, stirring vigorously to fully incorporate. Season with salt and pepper and stir to combine. Dressing will be creamy. Set aside. While not necessary, the dressing can be made a day ahead of time to allow flavors to develop more thoroughly.

3. To prepare the salad, use the same pan that toasted the curry powder to toast pistachios over medium heat until fragrant or toast marks start to show, 1 to 2 minutes. Transfer to a small bowl, and set aside to cool. Add the baby greens, cucumber, carrot, red onion, and banana to a large bowl. Top with toasted pistachios. Using a spatula, add dressing to salad to coat. It may be helpful to toss by hand, wearing plastic gloves to reduce mess. Garnish with remaining banana slices if desired.

Nutrition: 230 calories, 18 g total fat, 2 g saturated fat, 3 g protein, 18 g carbohydrates, 4 g fiber

Salmon and Blueberry Salad with Red Onion Vinaigrette

Warm salmon, red onions, and blueberries make a sweet and savory pairing in this salad. It's perfect for lunch or dinner.

MIND foods: Olive oil, fish, leafy greens, berries

Yield: 4 servings

Time: 35 minutes to prep; 25 minutes to cook

Difficulty: Easy

1 medium red onion, thinly sliced in half rings

¼ cup red wine vinegar

1 teaspoon sugar

1 teaspoon salt, divided

¼ teaspoon pepper, divided

3 tablespoons extra-virgin olive oil, divided

1½ pounds salmon fillets, cut crosswise in 4 portions

6 cups lettuce leaves, torn into bite-size pieces

1 cup fresh blueberries

1. In a microwaveable cup, combine onion, red wine vinegar, ½ teaspoon of the salt, and ⅛ teaspoon of the pepper; cover loosely with plastic wrap and microwave on high for 1 minute. Let stand, stirring occasionally, until onions turn pink, about 15 minutes.

2. Meanwhile, preheat grill or broiler. Brush 1 tablespoon of the olive oil on both sides of the salmon fillets; sprinkle with remaining ½ teaspoon of salt and ⅛ teaspoon of pepper. Grill or broil salmon, skin side down, until just cooked through, about 6 minutes. Divide lettuce leaves among four dinner plates and place salmon in the center. With a slotted spoon, remove onions from vinegar; scatter onions, along with the blueberries, over and around the fish. Whisk remaining 2 tablespoons of the olive oil into the vinegar mixture. Drizzle vinaigrette over salmon.

Nutrition: 290 calories, 16 g total fat, 2 g saturated fat, 30 g protein, 6 g carbohydrates, 1 g fiber

Recipe courtesy of U.S. Highbush Blueberry Council | www.littlebluedynamos.com

Blueberry, Peach, and Avocado Salad

Basil and lime juice bring bright flavor to this fruit salad. Creamy avocado adds a savory twist, making it a perfect snack for any time of day.

MIND foods: Olive oil, berries

Yield: 6 servings

Time: 20 to 25 minutes

Difficulty: Easy

> 1 tablespoon extra-virgin olive oil
>
> 1 tablespoon lime juice
>
> ½ teaspoon lime zest
>
> ¼ teaspoon salt
>
> 2 cups fresh blueberries
>
> 2 large ripe peaches, pitted and cubed
>
> 1 avocado, pitted and cubed
>
> 1 tablespoon finely chopped fresh basil

3. In a large bowl whisk olive oil, lime juice, lime zest, and salt until well blended. Add blueberries, peaches, avocado, and basil. Toss gently to combine. Serve.

Nutrition: 130 calories, 8 g total fat, 1 g saturated fat, 1.5 g protein, 16 g carbohydrates, 4 g fiber

Recipe courtesy of U.S. Highbush Blueberry Council | www.littlebluedynamos.com

Pomegranate Avocado Quinoa Grain Salad

This salad is perfect for the cooler months when pomegranates and avocados are at their best. Combined with hearty greens and pecans, it's like a one-dish meal. Pair it with a veggie-rich soup for a simple, easy dinner.

MIND foods: Whole grains, berries, nuts, leafy greens, olive oil

Yield: 4 servings

Time: 10 minutes to prep; 50 minutes to cook

Difficulty: Easy

> 2 cups cooked quinoa, cooled (can be made ahead)
>
> 1 cup pomegranate arils (seeds)
>
> ¼ cup chopped pecans
>
> 1 avocado, diced
>
> 2 cups chopped fresh greens (kale, chard, or spinach)
>
> ¼ cup chopped fresh basil
>
> 1 lime, juiced
>
> 1 tablespoon extra-virgin olive oil
>
> 1 tablespoon pomegranate molasses
>
> 2 cloves garlic, minced
>
> ¼ teaspoon pepper
>
> Pinch sea salt (optional)

1. Combine quinoa, pomegranate, pecans, avocado, greens, and basil in a medium bowl. In a small bowl, whisk together lime juice, oil, pomegranate molasses, garlic, pepper, and sea salt. Pour dressing over salad, combine well, and serve immediately.

Nutrition: 320 calories, 16 g total fat, 2 g saturated fat, 7 g protein, 40 g carbohydrates, 8 g fiber

Recipe by Sharon Palmer, RDN | www.sharonpalmer.com

Salmon Lentil Barley Grain Salad

This delicious salad was developed in celebration for Wear Red Day, which was created by the American Heart Association to promote awareness about heart disease and stroke among women. While this is considered a heart-healthy recipe, it's also perfect for the MIND diet. Remember: if it is good for the heart, then it is good for the brain.

MIND foods: Fish, whole grains, leafy greens, berries, olive oil

Yield: 1 serving, including 1 tablespoon of dressing (there will be leftover dressing)

Time: 10 minutes to prep; 50 minutes to cook

Difficulty: Medium

> 4-ounce salmon fillet
>
> Salt and pepper, to taste
>
> ½ cup lentils
>
> ½ cup barley
>
> 1 teaspoon extra-virgin olive oil
>
> ½ cup spinach and microgreens
>
> ½ orange, segmented
>
> 1 tablespoon pomegranate arils
>
> 2 tablespoons toasted hemp seeds and pepitas

Dressing:

> 2–3 tablespoons fresh-squeezed orange juice
>
> 2 tablespoons plus 1 teaspoon tahini
>
> 2 tablespoons apple cider vinegar
>
> 1 tablespoon maple syrup
>
> 1 tablespoon extra-virgin olive oil

1. Preheat oven to 350°F. Heat two small pots of water on medium-high heat. Pat salmon dry with paper towels then rub with salt and pepper on both sides. Let rest at room temperature while preparing other ingredients.

2. When water is boiling, add lentils to one pot and barley to the other. Lentils will need 25 minutes; barley will need 45 minutes. While barley and lentils are cooking, place salmon skin side down on a baking sheet and drizzle with olive oil. Bake until the fish is flaky, about 20 minutes. To check, take a fork and see

if the fish will flake easily. The low temperature will keep the salmon moist.

3. While salmon, lentils, and barley are cooking, prepare the dressing by combining all ingredients and whisking together. Drain barley and lentils when the time is up for each, then combine in a large bowl and set aside. Once salmon is cooked, flake and add it to the large bowl. Add all remaining ingredients, except for dressing, and gently combine. Plate your meal and drizzle with 1 tablespoon of dressing—you will have leftovers of the delicious dressing.

Nutrition: 530 calories, 15 g total fat, 2 g saturated fat, 35 g protein, 60 g carbohydrates, 15 g fiber

Recipe by Margot Witteveen, MS, RDN, LD | www.silverspoonsnutrition.co

Sorghum Pomegranate Tabbouleh Grain Salad

This easy-to-make tabbouleh uses sorghum, which is a gluten-free grain that's a source of protein. Jewel-like pomegranate adds antioxidants and crunch to the dish.

MIND foods: Whole grains, olive oil, berries

Yield: 4 servings

Time: 15 minutes to prep; 1 hour to cook

Difficulty: Easy

1 cup sorghum kernels

3 cups water

1 garlic clove, minced

¼ teaspoon salt

2 tablespoons extra-virgin olive oil

4 cups curly leaf parsley

¼ cup fresh mint, torn into small pieces

½ pomegranate arils

1. In a large saucepan, bring the sorghum and water to a boil. Reduce heat and simmer until the sorghum is tender, about 1 hour. Place the cooled sorghum in a large bowl and add the garlic, salt, and olive oil, tossing to coat. While sorghum is cooking, pulse the parsley in a blender until coarsely chopped. Add the parsley, mint, and pomegranate to the sorghum mixture and toss to combine.

Nutrition: 260 calories, 9 g total fat, 1 g saturated fat, 8 g protein, 44 g carbohydrates, 6 g fiber

Recipe by Abby Langer, RD | www.abbylangernutrition.com

Farro-Cabbage Grain Salad

This salad is filling and flavorful thanks to the farro and a spice-filled dressing. Cabbage adds crunch. For a different flavor, substitute packaged broccoli slaw for the cabbage.

MIND foods: Leafy greens, whole grains, olive oil

Yield: 4 servings

Time: 30 minutes

Difficulty: Easy

2½ cups shredded red or white cabbage

2 cups cooked farro (cooked according to package directions)

3 scallions, sliced

½ cup chopped fresh parsley

3 tablespoons orange juice

1½ tablespoons extra-virgin olive oil

1 clove garlic, minced

¼ teaspoon red pepper flakes

½ teaspoon ground cumin

½ teaspoon chili powder

¼ teaspoon ground turmeric

1. In a large bowl, toss together the cabbage, farro, scallions, and parsley. In a small bowl, whisk together the orange juice, olive oil, garlic, red pepper flakes, cumin, chili powder, and turmeric to make the dressing. Pour the dressing on the salad, toss, and serve.

Nutrition: 230 calories, 6 g total fat, 1 g saturated fat, 8 g protein, 38 g carbohydrates, 6 g fiber

Recipe courtesy of Oldways Whole Grains Council | www.oldwayspt.org, www.wholegrainscouncil.org

Berry Gazpacho Soup

The hot days of summer are perfect for a chilled gazpacho soup, and nothing says summer like berries.

MIND foods: Wine, berries

Yield: 4 servings

Time: 45 minutes, plus 4 to 6 hours of chill time

Difficulty: Medium

Gazpacho:

1 bottle Riesling wine

1 bunch fresh mint

1 sprig basil

3 cups strawberries, halved

Zest and juice of 1 large lemon

Finishing:

4 teaspoons toasted almond slices

½ cup blueberries

4 teaspoons extra-virgin olive oil, for garnish

Pinch pepper

Pinch pink Himalayan salt

1. In a medium saucepan, combine the wine, mint, and basil, and bring to a boil. Reduce heat and let simmer until reduced by half.

2. Meanwhile, toast almond slices in a small pan over low to medium heat until color begins to change and almonds are fragrant, about 2 to 3 minutes. Set aside.

3. When wine mixture has reduced by half, carefully discard mint and basil before adding strawberries, lemon zest, and lemon juice to the saucepan. Cook for 5 minutes to soften berries. Using an immersion blender, puree ingredients together until smooth. Cook for another 5 minutes. Remove from heat and let cool for 15 minutes. Transfer to storage containers and refrigerate until completely cold, 4 to 6 hours.

4. When ready to serve, share among four bowls and evenly distribute toppings of blueberries and toasted almond slices. Drizzle each bowl with a teaspoon of olive oil, and a pinch of pink salt and pepper.

Nutrition: 260 calories, 6 g total fat, 1 g saturated fat, 2 g protein, 17 g carbohydrates, 3 g fiber

Quick Chicken-Tortilla Soup

This is a quick and easy recipe that has all the flavors of a Sonoran Mexican classic soup. Although the ingredient list appears long, it's the seasonings and toppers that lengthen it. Nothing fancy going on here, just a combination of fresh ingredients and pantry staples. Using fresh and canned vegetables, this flavorful and healthy dish is a feast for the eyes and the taste buds.

MIND foods: Olive oil, vegetables, poultry, whole grains

Yield: 6 servings

Time: 10 to 15 minutes to prep; 20 minutes to cook

Difficulty: Easy

2 teaspoons extra-virgin olive oil

1 cup yellow or sweet onion, chopped

1 jalapeño pepper, seeded and chopped (optional)

1 (4-ounce) can mild green chilies

3 medium tomatoes, cored and chopped

2 garlic cloves, chopped and smashed

1 tablespoon tomato paste

1 tablespoon ground cumin

1 teaspoon ground coriander

¼ teaspoon dried Mexican oregano

6 cups low-sodium chicken stock or broth

1 pound chicken, cooked and shredded (this recipe uses store-bought rotisserie chicken)

⅓ cup (or more) fresh cilantro leaves, plus more to top (optional)

2 tablespoons freshly squeezed lime juice, plus more to top (optional)

⅛ teaspoon salt

¼ teaspoon pepper

Tortilla strips:

6 corn tortillas

canola oil spray

Optional soup toppers:

1 avocado, peeled, seeded, and diced

½ cup reduced-fat sour cream or plain Greek yogurt

1. Preheat oven to 350°F. In a large pot, heat oil over medium heat. Add onion, jalapeño, green chilies, and sauté for a few minutes. Add tomatoes and garlic and stir to combine. Add tomato paste

to the pot and allow the paste to melt into the other ingredients for about one minute. Add cumin, coriander, and oregano and stir to combine. Increase heat and add broth, then add chicken. Bring soup to a boil then simmer for about 10 minutes. Add cilantro, lime juice, salt and pepper. Stir well. Remove soup from heat and cover to keep warm.

2. To prepare tortilla strips, stack 3 corn tortillas and slice into ½-inch-wide strips. Repeat process. Lay strips on a foil-lined baking sheet, spray with canola oil, and place into oven. Bake for 10 to 15 minutes or until golden. Be careful not to burn the strips! Ladle soup into bowls and top with baked tortilla strips and optional toppers, including avocado, sour cream or yogurt, extra lime juice, and (my favorite) more cilantro!

Nutrition: 200 calories, 8 g total fat, 2 g saturated fat, 26 g protein, 8 g carbohydrates, 1.5 g fiber

Recipe by Christy Wilson, RDN | www.christywilsonnutrition.com

Red Lentil and Sweet Potato Soup

When the weather turns chilly, what better way to warm up than with a comforting bowl of soup? This red lentil soup is perfect for these types of occasions, and you'll love how easy it is to make. The best part of this recipe is that with all of the nutrients and large flavors present, it's sure to be a huge hit with your friends and family. Thanks to the sweet potatoes, this recipe is packed full of potassium, magnesium, iron, calcium, and manganese, and contains 400 percent of the daily recommended value for vitamin A. Now that's something to celebrate.

MIND foods: Olive oil, vegetables

Yield: 9 (1-cup) servings

Time: 5 minutes to prep; 30 minutes to cook

Difficulty: Easy

2 tablespoons extra-virgin olive oil

1 teaspoon ground cumin

¼ teaspoon ground ginger or ½ teaspoon grated ginger

1 tablespoon curry powder

1 yellow onion, diced

1 garlic clove, chopped

½ cup chopped carrots

2 sweet potatoes, medium diced (about 3 cups)

3 cups water

4 cups low-sodium vegetable broth

1½ cups split red lentils

Parsley, for garnish (optional)

1. Heat the oil in a soup pot over medium heat. Place the cumin, ginger, and curry powder in the olive oil and cook until fragrant, about 1 to 2 minutes. Add the onion and sauté until translucent. Add the garlic and continue to sauté until golden. Add the carrots and sweet potatoes to the soup pot, stirring periodically for 1 to 2 minutes, then add water, broth, and red lentils. Cover and bring mixture to a gentle boil. Once boiling, remove cover and continue to simmer for 25 minutes. Puree the soup with an immersion blender. You can also use a high-speed blender on low speed, or in a standard blender, as long as the soup is divided into batches (this will make it easier to blend). Serve. Garnish with parsley, if desired.

Nutrition: 180 calories, 4 g total fat, 1 g saturated fat, 8 g protein, 28 g carbohydrates, 5 g fiber

Recipe by Tracee Yablon Brenner, RD, CHHC | www.triadtowellness.com

Butternut Squash Curry-Ginger Soup

Gently sweet and spicy, this soup brings fall flavors to life. Packed with vitamin A, fiber, and the zing of fresh ginger, it is sure to be one of your healthy favorites soon.

MIND foods: Olive oil, vegetables, beans (tofu)

Yield: 4 servings

Time: 8 minutes to prep; 22 minutes to cook

Difficulty: Easy

> 2 teaspoons extra-virgin olive oil
>
> 1 small yellow onion, diced
>
> 1-inch ginger root, peeled and minced (reserve a pinch for garnish)
>
> 4 garlic cloves, minced
>
> 2 teaspoons toasted garam masala curry powder
>
> 4 cups peeled and cubed butternut squash
>
> 4 cups chicken or vegetable broth
>
> 1 cup soft tofu
>
> 2 teaspoons chopped fresh parsley
>
> Salt and pepper, to taste

1. In a large pot, heat oil over medium heat. Add the onion and sweat until translucent, then season with salt and pepper. Add ginger root and garlic cloves and sauté until fragrant, about 1 minute. Stir in curry powder. Add butternut squash and broth, and bring soup to a boil. Reduce heat and simmer for 20 minutes or until squash is tender. Add tofu. Use an immersion blender to puree soup until very smooth. Season with salt and pepper. Serve hot, garnishing with fresh parsley and fresh ginger.

Nutrition: 150 calories, 5 g total fat, 1 g saturated fat, 7 g protein, 21 g carbohydrates, 3 g fiber

White Bean and Whole Grain Pasta Soup

This healthy, hearty soup will warm you up on a cool day. The earthy yet delicate white beans pair with the complex whole grain texture and flavor of whole grain pasta. There's plenty to bite into here, making this soup a side dish that also works as a meal.

MIND foods: Olive oil, vegetables, beans, whole grains

Yield: 6 servings

Time: 10 minutes to prep; 35 minutes to cook

Difficulty: Easy

> 2 tablespoons plus 6 teaspoons extra-virgin olive oil, divided
>
> 1 large yellow onion, chopped
>
> Salt and pepper, to taste
>
> 3 large carrots, chopped
>
> 3 large celery stalks, chopped
>
> 1 head cauliflower, core removed, chopped into rice consistency
>
> 2 cups vegetable broth
>
> 2 cups water
>
> 1 (15-ounce) can navy beans, drained and rinsed
>
> ½ cup dry whole wheat (small shape) pasta
>
> 1 lemon, juiced
>
> Coarse sea salt

1. In a large soup pot, heat olive oil over medium heat until hot. Add onion and season with salt and pepper. Sauté until wilted and aromatic. Add carrots, celery, and cauliflower. Stir to coat all vegetables with olive oil and soften, 3 to 5 minutes. Add vegetable broth, water, and beans, and bring to a boil. Reduce heat to simmer for 25 minutes, stirring occasionally. Bring back up to a boil and add pasta, cooking until pasta is al dente, 6 to 8

minutes depending on the pasta type. Just before serving, drizzle each bowl with a teaspoon of olive oil, freshly squeezed lemon juice, and a very small pinch of coarse salt.

Nutrition: 320 calories, 15 g total fat, 2 g saturated fat, 11 g protein, 41 g carbohydrates, 10 g fiber

Snacks, Sides, & Spreads

Lemon Roasted Asparagus

Asparagus is a low-calorie, vitamin-rich, and fiber-dense vegetable. It is the perfect complement to the Mustard-Dill Crusted Salmon (page 178).

MIND foods: Vegetables, olive oil

Yield: 4 servings

Time: 5 minutes to prep; 10 to 12 minutes to cook

Difficulty: Easy

> 1 bunch of asparagus, bottom 2 inches trimmed
>
> 1 tablespoon extra-virgin olive oil
>
> 1 teaspoon freshly grated lemon zest
>
> Salt and pepper, to taste
>
> Lemon juice, to garnish

1. Preheat oven to 400°F. Toss asparagus with olive oil, lemon zest, and salt and pepper. Place on a sheet pan in a single layer. Roast in the oven for 10 to 12 minutes. Season with a fresh squeeze of lemon after removing from oven.

Nutrition: 50 calories, 4 g total fat, 1 g saturated fat, 2 g protein, 3 g carbohydrates, 1 g fiber

Recipe by Chef Allison Schaff, MS, RD, LD | www.prepdish.com

Collard Greens with Mustard Seeds

Collard greens are a nutritious, calcium-rich cruciferous vegetable that is packed with vitamins A and C. This recipe combines collard greens with flavorful apple cider vinegar, mustard seeds, and olive oil.

MIND foods: Olive oil, leafy greens

Yield: 4 servings

Time: 8 minutes to prep; 15 minutes to cook

Difficulty: Easy

> 2 tablespoons extra-virgin olive oil
>
> 1 small yellow onion, sliced
>
> 1 garlic clove, minced
>
> 1 tablespoon mustard seeds
>
> 1 bunch collard greens, sliced into ribbons
>
> 2 tablespoons apple cider vinegar
>
> 2 tablespoons water

1. In a medium sauté pan, add olive oil and onions, and sauté for about 5 minutes. Then add the garlic and sauté until light brown. Add the mustard seeds to the onion and garlic mixture, and shake them in the pan until they pop, about a minute or so. Place collard greens in sauté pan then add apple cider vinegar and water. Cover for 7 to 10 minutes. Serve immediately.

Nutrition: 75 calories, 7 g total fat, 1 g saturated fat, 1 g protein, 3 g carbohydrates, 1 g fiber

Recipe by Tracee Yablon Brenner, RD, CHHC | www.triadtowellness.com

Garlic Baby Bok Choy

This quick and simple vegetable side lets the quality and flavor of its few wholesome ingredients shine.

MIND diet foods: Leafy greens, olive oil

Yield: 2 servings

Time: 5 minutes to prep; 5 minutes to cook

Difficulty: Easy

> 1 teaspoon extra-virgin olive oil
>
> 3 garlic cloves, minced
>
> 1 bunch baby bok choy, rinsed, separated, and dried
>
> Salt and pepper, to taste

1. Heat olive oil in a nonstick skillet over low heat, add garlic, and sauté until fragrant. Avoid over-browning or burning the garlic pieces. Using a slotted spoon, remove garlic from oil and set aside. Add bok choy and small amount of salt and pepper, sautéing to coat in olive oil and evenly distribute spices. Cook to desired doneness or until leaves soften and wilt, about 3 minutes. Remove from heat. Add garlic back in and combine before serving.

Nutrition: 80 calories, 3 g total fat, 0 g saturated fat, 7 g protein, 11 g carbohydrates, 4 g fiber

Roasted Brussels Sprouts

Every healthy cook should have a foolproof way to enjoy Brussels sprouts. Roasting is one of the best ways to draw out the natural sweetness and reduce the bitterness of these cruciferous vegetables without compromising their hearty texture. Smaller, younger Brussels sprouts work best for this recipe.

MIND foods: Vegetables, olive oil

Yield: 6 servings

Time: 45 minutes

Difficulty: Easy

> 3 cups Brussels sprouts, trimmed and halved
>
> 2 large sweet onions, coarsely chopped
>
> 1 clove garlic, minced
>
> ¼ cup extra-virgin olive oil
>
> 1 lemon, juiced
>
> Salt and pepper, to taste

1. Preheat oven to 450°F. In a large bowl, combine all ingredients, mixing to coat Brussels sprouts and onions well. Spread onto a large baking sheet. Roast in oven for 20 to 25 minutes, stirring halfway through to rotate.

Nutrition: 120 calories, 9 g total fat, 1 g saturated fat, 2 g protein, 8 g carbohydrates, 2 g fiber

Oat Cranberry Pilaf with Pistachios

As a result of a challenge from the Cranberry Institute to create a holiday dish featuring oats, cranberries, pistachios, and turmeric, recipe contributor Sharon Palmer came up with this super-simple, plant-based side dish that involves one pan and a short list of ingredients. It's simple, nutritious, and flavorful.

MIND foods: Olive oil, vegetables, nuts, berries, whole grains

Yield: 8 servings

Time: 7 minutes to prep; 33 minutes to cook

Difficulty: Easy

1 teaspoon extra-virgin olive oil

1 small yellow onion, diced

3 stalks celery with leaves, diced

1 clove garlic, minced

½ cup chopped mushrooms

2 tablespoons chopped fresh parsley

¼ teaspoon ground turmeric

1 teaspoon ground marjoram

½ teaspoon pepper

⅓ cup pistachios, shelled

1 cup canned whole cranberries

2 cups vegetable broth

1½ cups old-fashioned oats

1. Heat oil in a large cast-iron skillet. Add onion, celery, and garlic, and sauté for 5 minutes. Add mushrooms, parsley, turmeric, marjoram, pepper, and pistachios, and sauté for an additional 3 minutes. While vegetables are cooking, heat oven to 350°F. Add cranberries, broth, and oats to the skillet, stirring until smooth. Transfer skillet to oven and bake on top rack for 25 minutes, until golden and tender.

Nutrition: 170 calories, 5 g total fat, 1 g saturated fat, 8 g protein, 26 g carbohydrates, 5 g fiber

Recipe by Sharon Palmer, RDN | www.sharonpalmer.com

Freekeh with Blueberries

This salad is as filling as it is delicious. Blueberries and freekeh make a perfect match with the addition of diverse flavors and herbs like chives and parsley. This salad is perfect as a side dish, or you can enjoy it for lunch. With fiber and protein, it will keep you full and ready to take on the day.

MIND foods: Whole grains, olive oil, berries, nuts

Yield: 4 servings

Time: 20 minutes to prep; 40 minutes to cook

Difficulty: Easy

 1 cup freekeh or farro

 2 cups chicken broth

 4 tablespoons extra-virgin olive oil

 3 tablespoons apple cider vinegar

 ¼ teaspoon salt

 ¼ teaspoon pepper

 ½ cup dried blueberries

 ½ cup fresh blueberries

 ½ cup chopped toasted shelled pistachios

 1 Fuji apple, cored and diced (can substitute any sweet red apple)

 ¼ cup chopped fresh parsley

 2 tablespoons snipped chives

1. In a medium skillet over medium-high heat, toast freekeh for 2 to 3 minutes, stirring until fragrant. Add the broth and bring to a boil. Reduce heat to low, cover, and let simmer 20 to 25 minutes or until all of the liquid has been absorbed. Remove from heat; let stand 10 minutes.

2. In the meantime, in a small bowl, combine oil, vinegar, salt, and pepper, and set aside. Transfer freekeh to a large bowl. Add dried and fresh blueberries, pistachios, apple, parsley, and chives. Pour vinaigrette over the mixture, stirring until combined.

Nutrition: 340 calories, 21 g total fat, 3 g saturated fat, 6 g protein, 32 g carbohydrates, 8 g fiber

Recipe courtesy of U.S. Highbush Blueberry Council | www.littlebluedynamos.com

Mediterranean Orange Wheat

Recipe contributor Sharon Palmer came up with this recipe after enjoying "Syrian Wheat Orange Salad" at a restaurant in Greece. After studying the ingredients and flavor profile, she tried to reproduce the bright citrus flavors, exotic spices, and crunchy grains and nuts that were so flavorful and satisfying. This is what she came up with.

MIND foods: Whole grains, vegetables, nuts, olive oil

Yield: 10 servings

Time: 15 minutes to prep; 15 minutes to cook (allow additional time to chill if possible)

Difficulty: Easy

    4 cups water

    2 cups fine bulgur

    2 medium oranges, peeled and chopped

    1 cucumber, chopped

    ½ cup pine nuts

    ½ cup roughly chopped fresh basil leaves

    1½ tablespoons extra-virgin olive oil

    1 lemon, juiced

    1 tablespoon pomegranate molasses

    2 cloves garlic, minced

    ¼ teaspoon ground allspice

    1 teaspoon ground cumin

    ¼ teaspoon cayenne pepper

    Salt, to taste

1. Place water in a medium pot, cover, and bring to a boil. Turn off heat, add bulgur, stir quickly, cover, and let sit for 7 minutes. Remove lid and fluff with a fork. Allow bulgur to cool. Mix cooled bulgur with oranges, cucumber, pine nuts, and basil leaves.

2. In a small dish, whisk together the olive oil, lemon juice, pomegranate molasses, garlic, allspice, cumin, cayenne pepper, and salt. Add dressing to the salad and mix to distribute. Adjust seasonings as needed. Chill until serving time.

Nutrition: 190 calories, 7 g total fat, 1 g saturated fat, 5 g protein, 29 g carbohydrates, 6 g fiber

Recipe by Sharon Palmer, RDN | www.sharonpalmer.com

Mediterranean-Style Watermelon-Pistachio-Mint Couscous

This salad is a sweet yet savory salad with fruit, nuts, and mint tossed over delicate whole grains. It's simple, yet elegant. You can cook the couscous while you are chopping the watermelon, pistachios, and mint and whisking together the salad dressing.

MIND foods: Whole grains, nuts, olive oil

Yield: 3 servings

Time: 15 minutes to prep; 5 minutes to combine; plus 20 minutes to chill

Difficulty: Easy

½ cup whole wheat couscous

1 cup low-sodium vegetable broth

1 cup cubed watermelon

30 pistachios, shelled, lightly salted, and chopped

4 leaves fresh mint, coarsely chopped

Dressing:

2 tablespoons extra-virgin olive oil

1 tablespoon red wine vinegar (or any vinegar you prefer)

1 teaspoon Dijon mustard

½ teaspoon honey

Dash salt and pepper

1. On the stovetop, put couscous into a pot with broth. Bring to a boil, stir, turn off heat, and cover for 5 to 10 minutes to allow the liquid to absorb (couscous will continue cooking). Flake with a fork and allow to cool. Put cooled couscous in a medium bowl, and top with watermelon, pistachios, and mint. Whisk dressing ingredients together and drizzle over couscous mixture. Serve and enjoy.

Nutrition: 280 calories, 15 g total fat, 2 g saturated fat, 5 g protein, 30 g carbohydrates, 2 g fiber

Recipe by Vicki Shanta Retelny, RDN, LDN | www.simplecravingsrealfood.com

Fiesta Quinoa

This colorful side salad looks beautiful presented on a bed of leafy baby greens or served with whole grain tortilla chips for an appetizer. This recipe is flexible, so add or change the ingredients to what you like. Add edamame or shredded chicken for a main dish salad. In season, fresh tomatoes are a great addition too.

MIND foods: Whole grains, vegetables, beans, olive oil

Yield: 6 servings

Time: 10 minutes to prep; 20 minutes to cook; plus 30 minutes to chill

Difficulty: Easy

 1 cup quinoa

 2 cups vegetable broth

 2 ears corn, roasted and cut off cob

 1 red bell pepper, roasted and chopped

 1 (15-ounce) can black beans, rinsed and drained

 3 scallions, sliced

 ½ cup chopped cilantro

 3 limes, juiced

 2 tablespoons extra-virgin olive oil

1 teaspoon ground cumin

½ teaspoon salt

¼ teaspoon pepper

⅛ teaspoon cayenne pepper

1. Put quinoa and broth in a medium saucepan. Bring to a boil, cover, and simmer for 15 minutes or until tender. In a large bowl, mix together the quinoa, corn, bell pepper, beans, scallions, and cilantro. In a small bowl, whisk together lime juice, olive oil, and seasonings. Pour dressing over quinoa mixture. Cover and chill for at least 30 minutes to let flavors set.

Nutrition: 240 calories, 7 g total fat, 1 g saturated fat, 9 g protein, 37 g carbohydrates, 6 g fiber

Recipe courtesy of Oldways Whole Grains Council | www.oldwayspt.org, www.wholegrainscouncil.org

Amaranth with Peppers and Cabbage

This Latin American Heritage dish is a delicious way to utilize cabbage, a favorite winter vegetable. The mild heat from the poblano peppers perfectly complements the peppery amaranth grains, but feel free to substitute bell peppers if you prefer.

MIND foods: Whole grains, vegetables, olive oil, leafy greens

Yield: 4 servings

Time: 1½ hours

Difficulty: Easy

2 cups water

1 cup amaranth grains

2 garlic cloves, minced

1 green bell pepper, cored, seeded, and diced

1 poblano pepper (or substitute another bell pepper), cored, seeded, and diced

2 tablespoons extra-virgin olive oil

¼ head purple cabbage, chopped into long shreds

Salt and pepper, to taste

1. To cook the amaranth, bring the water and amaranth to a boil, then simmer, partially covered, for 30 to 35 minutes until soft, swollen, and tender. Remove from the heat and allow to stand for 15 minutes, with the lid still on, to swell more.

2. Meanwhile, in a large shallow pan over low to medium heat, gently sauté the garlic and diced pepper in the oil until the vegetables are soft. Add the cabbage, season with salt and pepper, and put the lid on to cook for 5 more minutes. Gently stir in the amaranth grains, reheat, and serve.

Nutrition: 270 calories, 11 g total fat, 1.5 g saturated fat, 8 g protein, 38 g carbohydrates, 6 g fiber

Recipe courtesy of Oldways Whole Grains Council | www.oldwayspt.org, www.wholegrainscouncil.org

Steel-Cut Oat Risotto with Mushrooms

Unlike some grains, which must be furiously stirred into submission, steel-cut oats give up their creaminess almost willingly, making them an ideal star for whole grain risotto. This rustic dish pairs exceptionally well with seafood.

MIND foods: Olive oil, vegetables, whole grains

Yield: 4 servings

Time: 10 minutes to prep; 35 minutes to cook

Difficulty: Medium

3 cups low-sodium vegetable broth

½ cup white wine

1 tablespoon extra-virgin olive oil

1 small yellow onion, chopped

2 garlic cloves, minced

1½ cups sliced white (button) mushrooms

1 cup dry steel-cut oats

Salt and pepper, to taste

2 tablespoons chopped fresh sage

1. Heat the broth and wine in a small pot over low to medium heat until warm, but not boiling. While the broth mixture is warming, heat the oil in a large pot over medium heat, then add the onion and cook for about 3 minutes, stirring occasionally. Add the garlic and mushrooms to the onions and cook for an additional minute. Stir the oats into the vegetable mixture, and add ½ cup of the warm broth mixture into the pot. Stir frequently over medium heat until all of the moisture is absorbed. Repeat, adding ½ cup of the broth mixture at a time, until all of the broth mixture is used and the oats reach a creamy consistency, approximately 20 to 25 minutes. Add salt and pepper, taste, and adjust seasonings. Divide the risotto into four bowls and garnish with fresh sage.

Nutrition: 250 calories, 6 g total fat, 1 g saturated fat, 8 g protein, 35 g carbohydrates, 6 g fiber

Recipe courtesy of Oldways Whole Grains Council, adapted from Sharon Palmer, RDN | www.oldwayspt.org, www.wholegrainscouncil.org

Guacamole-Stuffed Tomato Poppers

These poppers are the perfect party pleasers. They are so much fun to eat, and when you pop one in your mouth, a creamy flavorful burst explodes. It's hard to believe you get 6 grams of fiber from a serving of these creamy babies. And the fat is coming from the "good-for-you fats" in the avocado. The toughest part is not eating them all yourself. The recipe is fairly easy, but it takes a little skill and patience to stuff the guac in the poppers.

MIND foods: Vegetables

Yield: 4 servings (5 tomatoes per serving)

Time: 20 minutes

Difficulty: Medium

> **20 cherry tomatoes**
>
> **1 avocado, seeded and mashed**
>
> **1 lime, juiced**
>
> **1 garlic clove, mashed**
>
> **1 tablespoon cilantro, chopped (optional)**
>
> **1 small mango, small diced**

1. Wash cherry tomatoes and cut tops off. Carefully cut a sliver off the bottom to help them stand up. Be careful not to cut too deep or it'll make an opening on the bottom. Using a melon baller or knife, scoop out the insides until hollow. In a bowl, mix together mashed avocado, lime juice, garlic, and cilantro. Cut mango into tiny cubes so they will fit nicely in the cherry tomatoes. Gently stuff tomatoes with guacamole, top with mango, and serve as a healthy snack.

Nutrition: 190 calories, 8 g total fat, 1 g saturated fat, 4 g protein, 30 g carbohydrates, 6 g fiber

Recipe by Lyssie Lakatos and Tammy Lakatos Shames, RD, CDN, CFT, aka The Nutrition Twins® | www.NutritionTwins.com

Yucatan Beans with Pumpkin Seeds

This appetizer is very easy to toss together and is a perfect example of the great potential of canned beans. Pumpkin seeds and lime juice together add an unusual but delicious flavor. Serve alone as a bean salad, with crackers or bread, or on a bed of lettuce.

MIND foods: Vegetables, beans

Yield: 8 servings

Time: 15 minutes

Difficulty: Easy

¼ cup hulled pumpkin seeds (pepitas)

1 (15-ounce) can white beans, rinsed and drained

1 tomato, finely chopped

⅓ cup finely chopped white, yellow, or red onion

⅓ cup finely chopped cilantro

3–4 tablespoons lime juice

Salt and pepper, to taste

1. Toast the pumpkin seeds in a small skillet over medium heat, shaking the pan often, for 3 minutes, or until lightly browned. Transfer to a bowl to cool. Coarsely chop pumpkin seeds in a food processor or with a sharp knife. In a medium serving bowl, combine the pumpkin seeds, beans, tomato, onion, cilantro, and lime juice. Season with salt and pepper. Toss to combine. Season with more salt and lime juice, if desired.

Nutrition: 90 calories, 2 g total fat, 0 g saturated fat, 5 g protein, 12 g carbohydrates, 3 g fiber

Recipe courtesy of Oldways, adapted from chef Steven Raichlen | www.oldwayspt.org

Warm Rosemary Pistachios

A little warmth and fragrant rosemary bring the delicate buttery flavors in pistachios to a new level. This recipe is so simple, yet transforms pistachios into an elevated snack, just like that.

MIND foods: Olive oil, nuts

Yield: 2 servings of about 25 pistachios each

Time: 1 minute to prep; 4 minutes to cook

Difficulty: Easy

1 tablespoon extra-virgin olive oil

2 tablespoons chopped fresh rosemary

1 ounce in-shell pistachios (about 49 nuts, or ½ cup)

Salt and pepper, to taste

1. Gently heat olive oil in a medium pan over low-medium heat. Add rosemary and stir until fragrant, 1 to 2 minutes. Add pistachios and continually stir or shake pan in a circular motion until pistachios are well-coated, 1 to 2 minutes. Sprinkle with a small pinch of salt and pepper if desired. Remove from heat. They are a special treat when enjoyed warm, but they taste just as good at room temperature.

Nutrition: 150 calories, 14 g total fat, 2 g saturated fat, 3 g protein, 5 g carbohydrates, 2 g fiber

Popped Sorghum

Popped sorghum is a popular snack in India. Like popcorn, most other grains have the same moisture-sealed hull and dense core that lead to popping when enough steam pressure builds up inside the kernel. Popping corn is probably the fluffiest, but sorghum comes in second (most other grains, while they can be "popped," result in something that is more aptly described as "puffed").

MIND foods: Whole grains, olive oil

Yield: 2 servings

Time: 2 minutes to prep; 6 minutes to cook

Difficulty: Easy

¼ cup dry sorghum, divided

1 teaspoon chili flakes

1 teaspoon lime zest

1 tablespoon extra-virgin olive oil

1. Place half of the sorghum in a clean brown paper bag, folding the top down to close the bag. Place the bag in a microwave with the folded side facing down. Heat on high for 3 minutes, but stay attentive as it may not need all 3 minutes. Remove from

microwave when there is more than 10 seconds between pops. Carefully empty into a large bowl. Repeat with remaining ⅛ cup of sorghum. Sprinkle chili flakes and lime zest on top of the popped sorghum, and gently move bowl in circular motion to distribute. Drizzle with olive oil. With plastic gloves on, gently combine until all ingredients are evenly distributed.

Nutrition: 140 calories, 8 g total fat, 1 g saturated fat, 3 g protein, 17 g carbohydrates, 2 g fiber

Basic Salsa

Salsa is one of the world's most versatile and best-loved foods. With fresh and zesty flavors that bring any dish alive, it is loved by nutrition experts because it uses naturally wholesome fruits and vegetables, adding flavor without an overload of salt, sugar, and saturated fat. Everyone should have one solid basic salsa in their repertoire. It goes with everything, is easy to make, and is an excellent place to get started.

MIND foods: Vegetables

Yield: 4 servings (¼ cup each)

Time: 10 minutes plus 1+ hour to chill (optional)

Difficulty: Easy

>   3 Roma tomatoes, diced
>
>   1 medium sweet onion, diced
>
>   ¼ cup chopped fresh cilantro, rinsed and pat dry with paper towels
>
>   3 limes, juiced
>
>   Salt and pepper, to taste

1.   Combine tomatoes, onion, cilantro, and lime juice. Add salt and pepper to taste, keeping in mind that flavor will develop over time.

Nutrition: 30 calories, 0 g total fat, 0 g saturated fat, 1 g protein, 8 g carbohydrates, 1 g fiber

Black Bean Salsa

Black bean salsa is a hearty take on salsa. It's less of a topping and more of a side dish, or even meal-sized when a larger portion is enjoyed.

MIND foods: Beans, whole grains

Yield: 5 servings (½ cup each)

Time: 10 to prep; 30+ minutes to rest in refrigerator

Difficulty: Easy

> 1 (15-ounce) can black beans, drained and rinsed
>
> 3 Roma tomatoes, diced
>
> ¼ cup red onion, diced
>
> 1 cup fresh, frozen, or canned sweet corn
>
> ⅛ teaspoon ground cumin
>
> ½ cup chopped fresh cilantro, rinsed and pat dry
>
> 2 green onions, chopped
>
> 1 lime, juiced
>
> Salt and pepper, to taste

1. In a large bowl, combine all of the ingredients and stir to mix flavors together well. Cover and let rest in the refrigerator for at least half an hour.

Nutrition: 150 calories, 1 g total fat, 0 g saturated fat, 8 g protein, 29 g carbohydrates, 6 g fiber

Roasted Garlic Spread

After roasting, garlic loses its sharp bite and transforms into something gentle and creamy. Roasted garlic is delicious on just about anything—whole grain baguette rounds, mixed into mashed potatoes, or used in salad dressings. An added bonus: your kitchen will fill with the most appetizing aromas.

MIND foods: Vegetables, olive oil

Yield: 32 servings (¼ bulb per serving)

Time: 1 hour 20 minutes

Difficulty: Easy

> *8 heads of garlic*
>
> *½ cup extra-virgin olive oil*
>
> *Salt and pepper, to taste (optional)*

1. Preheat oven to 400°F. Trim the top quarter off the top of each head (you should see now-flat tops of the garlic cloves within). Place a large sheet of foil in a rimmed baking sheet. Place garlic heads in center of foil, and drizzle olive oil over exposed garlic, allowing it to soak in and around the garlic cloves. Sprinkle with salt and pepper, if desired. Tightly wrap the foil, and place in hot oven for about an hour or until a knife can easily pierce the cloves. Remove from oven and let stand to cool. Once cool enough to handle, use fingers to press bulb from base so that the garlic cloves pop out into a small bowl. Mash with a spoon or fork.

Nutrition: 40 calories, 3 g total fat, 0 g saturated fat, 1 g protein, 3 g carbohydrates, 0 g fiber

Beverages & Desserts

Almond Milk

Almond milk is simple to make at home for a fresh taste and control over how many almonds go into the mix (most store-bought almond milks contain very little actual almond). Play around with the amount of almonds you use until you find a texture and taste you prefer. Or experiment with other nuts using the same methods here (e.g., hazelnuts, cashews).

MIND foods: Nuts

Yield: 4 servings

Time: 10 minutes plus overnight soaking and optional 1+ hour chilling time

Difficulty: Easy

   1 cup almonds, soaked overnight (can do ahead)

   4 cups water

   2 Medjool dates, pitted

   1 teaspoon vanilla or almond extract

   Pinch salt

1. Rinse and drain soaked almonds. Add all ingredients to a blender and pulse on high until very well combined. Strain through a cheesecloth over a large bowl, reserving the almond

pulp for use in baked goods, oatmeal, or smoothies. Repeat straining process if desired. Store in a jar with a lid (mason jars work well). Chill if desired. Shake before serving.

Nutrition: 20 calories, .5 g total fat, 0 g saturated fat, 1 g protein, 3 g carbohydrates, 0 g fiber

Oat Milk

Oat milk is a mild-tasting dairy alternative that is simple and affordable to make at home. Experiment with different amounts of water to get the consistency you prefer.

MIND foods: Whole grains

Yield: 4 servings

Time: 5 to 10 minutes plus 1 hour chilling time

Difficulty: Easy

> 4 cups water
>
> 1 cup quick-cooking oats (aka rolled, regular, instant, old-fashioned)
>
> 2 Medjool dates, pitted
>
> 1 teaspoon vanilla extract
>
> Pinch salt

1. Bring water to a simmer in a small pot, then add all ingredients to cook for 5 minutes. Blend all ingredients in food processor or blender until combined. Strain through a fine mesh sieve over a large bowl, reserving oat solids to use in smoothies, soups, or oatmeal. Repeat straining process if desired. Store in a jar with a lid (mason jars work well). Chill for at least an hour. Shake before serving.

Nutrition: 30 calories, .5 g total fat, 0 g saturated fat, 1 g protein, 5 g carbohydrates, 0 g fiber

Superfood Smoothie

Smoothies are one of the easiest ways to make fruits and vegetables accessible to even the pickiest eater. The term "superfood" doesn't have a technical meaning, but here it refers to nutrient-packed whole foods from the MIND diet healthy food groups. Use this recipe as a starter guide, then experiment with your own combinations. Choose a mild leafy green (otherwise it may come out too bitter). This particular recipe throws in chia and hemp seeds for an even bigger nutrient boost.

MIND foods: Nuts, leafy greens, vegetables, berries

Yield: 4 servings

Time: 15 minutes

Difficulty: Easy

> 2 tablespoons chia seeds
>
> 1 cup almond milk
>
> 2 cups baby kale
>
> ½ cup chopped carrots
>
> ¼ cup fresh or frozen blueberries
>
> ¼ cup fresh or frozen strawberries
>
> ¼ cup fresh or frozen raspberries
>
> 2 tablespoons almond butter
>
> 1 tablespoon hemp seeds
>
> ½ cup 100% pomegranate juice

1. In a medium bowl, combine chia seeds and almond milk, and stir well. Let bowl rest in refrigerator. Meanwhile, add remaining ingredients to food processor or blender and pulse until all ingredients are pureed and very smooth. Add chia almond milk combination (it should have a gel-like consistency) to puree and pulse again until well combined. Divide into four glasses and serve.

Nutrition: 170 calories, 8 g total fat, 1 g saturated fat, 5 g protein, 18 g carbohydrates, 5 g fiber

Raspberry Almond Oat Shake

Packed with antioxidants, heart-healthy fat, whole grains, and a major protein punch, this smoothie will start your day out strong, pick you up when you hit your mid-afternoon slump, or refuel your body after a workout. With 18 grams of fiber in this shake, you'll be taking care of more than 70 percent of the Daily Value for this important nutrient. This shake is hearty enough to be a meal, or can be split in half for a snack that's still substantial. Save the other half for later, or share with a friend.

MIND foods: Berries, whole grains, nuts

Yield: 1 serving

Time: 10 minutes

Difficulty: Easy

> 1 cup frozen raspberries
>
> ¾ cup low-fat milk or milk alternative
>
> 3 tablespoons dry oats
>
> 2 tablespoons almonds
>
> 1 tablespoon ground flaxseed

1. Combine all ingredients in a blender and blend until smooth. Pour into a glass and enjoy.

Nutrition: 490 calories, 29 g total fat, 3 g saturated fat, 21 g protein, 46 g carbohydrates, 18 g fiber

Recipe courtesy of National Processed Raspberry Council | www.redrazz.org

High-Protein Banana Chocolate Chip Breakfast Cookies

Who doesn't love a warm chocolate chip cookie? Instead of an option heavy with added sugar and refined flour, reach for a cookie packed full of whole grains, nutrient-rich ingredients, and protein. This recipe only takes minutes to make and even the biggest kitchen novice will be able to tackle it.

MIND foods: Whole grains

Yield: 18 servings

Time: 5 minutes to prep; 15 minutes to bake

Skill level: Easy

1 large banana, mashed

¾ cup low-fat vanilla Greek yogurt

1 egg

1 cup oat flour

¼ teaspoon vanilla

1 teaspoon baking powder

¼ teaspoon salt

½ cup dark chocolate chips

1. Preheat oven to 400°F and line a cookie sheet with parchment paper. In a large bowl, combine banana and Greek yogurt, and vanilla; mix well. Whisk egg in a medium bowl, then add to liquid ingredients. Fold in dry ingredients (everything but the chocolate chips) and mix well. Add in chocolate chips and mix until evenly distributed. Scoop dough by the tablespoon onto lined cookie sheets and bake for 15 to 18 minutes until edges are light brown. Serve warm or cooled and store leftovers in refrigerator.

Nutrition per serving: 60 calories, 1.5 g total fat, 0.5 g saturated fat, 3 g protein, 9 g carbohydrates, 2 g fiber

Recipe by Erin Palinski-Wade, RD, CDE | www.erinpalinski.com

Chia Pudding

Chia seeds on grocery shelves today are related to but not the same as the ones used to grow green hair on "chia pets" some years ago. The chia seed that has gained recent traction in the hearts and minds of the health-conscious eater is one that boasts more of the plant form of omega-3 fats (alpha-linolenic acid) than flaxseeds, and way more fiber than oatmeal. Seeds, like nuts, tend to be concentrated sources of nutrients, so it's no surprise that chia scores high in health-boosting nutrition. Add nuts and berries, and this is a nutritionist-approved pudding.

MIND foods: Nuts, beans, berries

Yield: 4 servings

Time: 15 minutes

Difficulty: Easy

> 1½ cups unsweetened almond milk
>
> ½ cup soft tofu
>
> ½ teaspoon almond or vanilla extract
>
> ¼ cup chia seeds
>
> ¼ cup sliced almonds
>
> 1 cup fresh blueberries

1. In a medium bowl, whisk almond milk, tofu, and extract until well combined. Add chia seeds, stir to combine, and let rest for 10 minutes. Meanwhile, heat small skillet to low-medium heat, add almond slices, and continuously stir or shake until lightly toasted. Remove from heat and set aside. Gently add blueberries to chia mixture. Distribute evenly into four small bowls, garnish with toasted almonds, and serve immediately. Alternatively, refrigerate chia pudding mixture and serve chilled. Just before serving, distribute and garnish as before.

Nutrition: 190 calories, 12 g total fat, 1 g saturated fat, 7 g protein, 16 g carbohydrates, 7 g fiber

Blueberry Banana Ice Cream

With only three ingredients and no ice cream machine necessary, this blueberry-banana "ice cream" is a quick and easy way to satisfy any sweet tooth—no added sugar required.

MIND foods: Berries

Yield: 4 servings

Time: 5 minutes plus 2 hours advance freezing time for bananas

Difficulty: Easy

> *2 frozen bananas, chopped*
>
> *1 cup frozen blueberries*
>
> *2 vanilla beans, split lengthwise*

1. Chop and peel bananas before freezing. Freeze for at least 2 hours. This can be done ahead of time.

2. Add bananas and blueberries into a powerful blender or food processor. Scrape vanilla seeds in from the beans and process or blend until creamy. Be sure to scrape down the bowl or pitcher to make sure all of the ingredients fully blend in for ultimate creaminess. Scoop into bowls and serve.

Nutrition: 140 calories, 1 g total fat, 0 g saturated fat, 2 g protein, 35 g carbohydrates, 5 g fiber

Recipe courtesy of U.S. Highbush Blueberry Council | www.littlebluedynamos.com

Chocolate Banana Raspberry Mousse

In minutes you can whip up a decadent, guilt-free dessert that will satisfy your chocolate craving without all the added sugar.

MIND foods: Nuts, berries

Yield: 2 servings

Time: 10 minutes

Difficulty: Easy

> 2 medium bananas
>
> ¼ cup unsweetened cocoa powder
>
> ¼ cup almond butter
>
> ⅓ cup frozen raspberries
>
> 2 dates, pitted

1. Put all ingredients in a food processor and blend until smooth. Spoon into bowls and serve immediately, or refrigerate and serve chilled.

Nutrition: 380 calories, 20 g total fat, 2.5 g saturated fat, 11 g protein, 51 g carbohydrates, 13 g fiber

Recipe courtesy of National Processed Raspberry Council | www.redrazz.org

PART FOUR
Tips & Tools

CHAPTER 8

A Brain-Healthy Lifestyle

A healthy diet and lifestyle have so many benefits. This chapter reviews recommendations from Alzheimer's disease experts and the National Institute on Aging.

The following seven diet and lifestyle guidelines to prevent Alzheimer's disease are the result of an expert panel meeting at the 2013 International Conference on Nutrition and the Brain in Washington, D.C. Notably, Dr. Martha Clare Morris, lead MIND diet researcher, helped put these guidelines together. They were published in the journal *Neurobiology of Aging* in 2014. The scientists dutifully note that the scientific evidence is not yet complete, and that they compiled these practical everyday guidelines using the precautionary principle (i.e., better safe than sorry), using the best evidence available to them. Here are the guidelines at a glance:

1. Avoid saturated and trans fat.

2. Most of what you eat should be vegetables, legumes, fruits, and whole grains.

3. Eat food, and not supplements, for vitamin E.

4. Find a good source of vitamin B12 every day.

5. If you take a multivitamin, skip the minerals, especially iron and copper.

6. Avoid aluminum, which can be in cookware, antacids, baking powder, and other products.

7. Walk briskly for 40 minutes every other day.

Many of the recommendations should look familiar, as they're in line with diet and lifestyle advice for the general public, such as eat more vegetables and exercise regularly. Other recommendations are more specific to the research on cognitive decline and Alzheimer's disease, such as avoid aluminum.

This book has covered guidelines one through four, and guideline seven is self-explanatory, so the below will briefly discuss guidelines five and six.

Guideline 5: Avoid multivitamins with iron and copper. Iron and copper are essential nutrients important for good health. However, some studies suggest that excessive intake of these minerals, especially in combination with a diet high in saturated fat, contributes to cognitive problems and increased risk of Alzheimer's disease. Multivitamins commonly contain high amounts of both iron and copper, even though most people in the United States meet recommended levels of these nutrients through food. Unless specifically guided by your physician, it's best to choose foods first, and if using a multivitamin, to choose one with vitamins only.

Guideline 6: Avoid aluminum. The role of aluminum in Alzheimer's disease is controversial. Some researchers call for caution, while most experts agree that there is not enough evidence to say it clearly increases the risk for Alzheimer's disease. Aluminum, at high enough levels, has known neurotoxic potential. Aluminum has been found in the brains of people with Alzheimer's disease, and studies in Europe have observed higher rates of Alzheimer's disease in areas where the tap water was higher in aluminum.

LIFESTYLE GUIDELINES TO IMPROVE HEALTH AND WELL-BEING

The National Institute on Aging (NIA) has more general lifestyle guidelines to improve overall health and well-being to lower the risk of conditions that may increase the risk of Alzheimer's disease, such as heart disease and diabetes.

- Healthy diet

- Physical activity

- Healthy weight

- No smoking

The NIA also recommends that older adults participate in activities for social engagement and mental stimulation. Here are some examples of positive social activities:

- Attend the theater or a sporting event.

- Travel with a group of friends.

- Visit family and friends.

- Serve meals at a soup kitchen.

- Volunteer at a local animal shelter, school, library, or hospital.

Stimulate your mind by doing some of these activities:

- Take a cooking, art, or computer class.

- Form or join a book club.

- Learn how to play a musical instrument.

- Play cards or other games with friends.

- Sing in a community choral group.

Aluminum has no role in human biology, so there is no downside to avoiding exposure. In an abundance of caution, exposure can be minimized until the science has progressed. Aluminum is in some brands of baking powder, antacids, hemorrhoid medication, and other over-the-counter medicines; boxed cake mixes; deodorants and antiperspirants; douches; processed cheese; pickles; toothpaste; and table salts. As a food additive, aluminum is used as a firming agent in pickled products, as a pH-adjusting part of baking powder in bakery products, as an emulsifying agents in processed cheese spread, and in food colorings. Look for it on the ingredients list of packaged items.

CHAPTER 9

Tip Sheets

Top 10 Practical Kitchen Shortcuts for Making the MIND Diet Easy

Cooking from fresh, whole foods is ideal. But when you don't have the time or foods are out of season, look to these great shortcuts to make the MIND diet even simpler to implement.

1. Frozen leafy green vegetables are available year-round.

2. Frozen other vegetables are available year-round.

3. For berries, look to maximize fresh intake when they're in season in the spring and summer; otherwise, buy frozen.

4. For nuts, buy in bulk. Separate into weekly allotments and freeze what you're not using and they'll last for six months or longer.

5. Canned or cartoned beans are a major time-saver; just be sure to rinse them before use to shed residue and as much sodium as possible. Better yet, look for low-sodium options. And, if able, choose BPA-free packaging.

6. Check out whole grains marketed as "10-minute" versions to cut down on prep time. Frozen grains reheat nicely, including red rice and quinoa.

7. Packaged, shelf-stable fish comes in pouches, cans, jars, and tubes. Commonly seen on the shelf: tuna, salmon, sardines, mackerel, and anchovies.

8. For poultry, it doesn't get much easier than picking up a rotisserie chicken at your local grocer for a time save.

9. Buy smaller bottles of good-quality extra-virgin olive oil to keep them fresher and preserve the polyphenols.

10. For wine, remember to drink what you prefer—that's the only rule. If you need help on where to start, popular, versatile wines are pinot noir for reds and chardonnay for whites.

Top 10 Untraditional Ways to Use MIND Foods

The MIND diet celebrates wholesome, natural, simple foods. That doesn't mean it has to be boring. On the contrary, here are 10 new ways to think about the classic foods in the MIND diet.

1. Black bean brownies are fudgy, delicious, and flourless. Pureed black beans replace flour and offer more phytonutrients and fiber. Stealth-health at its best. No one will ever guess the secret ingredient is black beans.

2. Leafy greens aren't just for salads; try them in smoothies. Blend them with your favorite frozen fruit and you may not even notice there's a vegetable in your glass; or, load up

on the leafy greens portion and combine with ginger and apples for a veggie-forward green juice.

3. Add silken soft tofu to smoothies and soups to make them rich and creamy without the cream. The mild flavor of tofu incorporates seamlessly into sweet and savory dishes alike. It'll also boost the plant protein in any meal.

4. Fish for breakfast may sound unusual, but give it a try. Mash an anchovy in extra-virgin olive oil and combine with diced tomatoes. Top toast.

5. Pop sorghum like popcorn. It'll pop into a soft white snack, slightly smaller than the popcorn you're used to. Wild rice, amaranth, quinoa, barley, wheat berries, and millet all pop, or at least puff.

6. Make cauliflower into rice or couscous by cutting a head of cauliflower into quarters, removing the hard core and stem, and chopping until the pieces are your preferred size of rice or couscous (or give it a rough chop and add the pieces into a food processor to blend briefly until the consistency you prefer is achieved). Heat for five to seven minutes with extra-virgin olive oil over medium heat, then mix in green veggies for a healthy side dish.

7. Grilled berries make for a decadent dessert with no added sugar. Simply choose your favorite berries and wrap them in a parchment-paper-lined sheet of foil, or try adding lemon zest and balsamic vinegar to your berry mix for more complex flavors. Grill for about five minutes.

8. Breakfast porridge or oatmeal works surprisingly well as a savory dish. Try steel-cut oats topped with kimchi, a poached egg, and green onions; or, enjoy with shredded chicken and your favorite salsa.

9. Use veggies instead of pasta. Spaghetti squash can step in for long spaghetti noodles, and long, flat slices of zucchini can stand in for lasagna pasta.

10. Add nut butters to smoothies and oatmeal for a rich, creamy flavor and up the protein and healthy fat content too.

Top 10 Plant Proteins

Plant proteins are affordable, sustainable, and delicious. Here are 10 great options to try, each with at least 5 grams of protein per serving.

1. Firm tofu—11 g per half cup

2. Hemp hearts—10 g per ounce

3. Kamut wheat—10 g per cup (cooked)

4. White beans—9 g per half cup (cooked)

5. Quinoa—8 g per cup (cooked)

6. Black beans—8 g per half cup (cooked)

7. Wild rice—7 g per cup (cooked)

8. Almonds—6 g per ounce

9. Pistachios—6 g per ounce

10. Buckwheat groats—6 g per cup (cooked)

Top 10 Sustainable Seafood Choices

Sustainable seafood is well-managed and caught or farmed in ways with minimal environmental harm to habitats or other wildlife. The options below have been vetted by the Monterey Bay Aquarium and are current as of 2016. For the most up-to-date information, contact them at www.seafoodwatch.org.

1. Arctic char (farmed)
2. Barramundi (US farmed, Vietnam farmed)
3. Clams, mussels, and oysters
4. Pacific cod (Alaska)
5. Sablefish (Alaska, Canada farmed)
6. Salmon (Alaska, New Zealand)
7. Pacific sardines (Canada, US)
8. Scallops (farmed)
9. Shrimp (US farmed, Alaska)
10. Rainbow trout (US farmed)

Top 10 Fiber-Rich Beans

Meeting daily fiber goals are much easier with beans on the menu. All beans are healthy choices and offer good nutrition. The beans on this list are excellent sources of fiber, providing at least 5 grams of fiber per half-cup cooked serving, or 20 percent of the Daily Value (25 grams) for fiber.

1. Navy beans—10 g fiber, 130 calories

2. Small white beans—9 g fiber, 130 calories

3. Cranberry (Roman) beans—9 g fiber, 130 calories

4. Chickpeas (garbanzo beans)—8 g fiber, 180 calories

5. Pinto beans—8 g fiber, 120 calories

6. Lima beans—7 g fiber, 110 calories

7. Great northern beans—6 g fiber, 150 calories

8. White beans—6 g fiber, 150 calories

9. Kidney beans—6 g fiber, 110 calories

10. Soybeans—5 g fiber, 150 calories

Top 10 Simple Snack Pairings

Eating doesn't have to be complicated. In fact, sometimes there's nothing nicer or more nutritious than the simplest of dishes. Here are 10 ideas for MIND-friendly snacks that are easy, healthy, and so delicious.

1. Fresh apricot with 49 pistachios

   MIND foods: Nuts

   Nutrition: 180 calories, 13 g total fat, 2 g saturated fat, 6 g protein, 12 g carbohydrates, 4 g fiber

2. Half-cup of halved strawberries with 23 almonds

   MIND foods: Berries, nuts

   Nutrition: 200 calories, 16 g total fat, 1 g saturated fat, 7 g protein, 11 g carbohydrates, 4 g fiber

3. A slice of 100 percent whole wheat toast topped with a quarter of a small California avocado, a squeeze of fresh lemon juice, and chili pepper flakes

   MIND foods: Whole grains

   Nutrition: 120 calories, 6 g total fat, 1 g saturated fat, 4 g protein, 14 g carbohydrates, 4 g fiber

4. 15 baby carrots drizzled with 2 teaspoons extra-virgin olive oil and 1 teaspoon balsamic vinegar, sprinkled with pepper

   MIND foods: Vegetables, olive oil

   Nutrition: 150 calories, 9 g total fat, 1 g saturated fat, 1 g protein, 15 g carbohydrates, 4 g fiber

5. Chopped ripe medium tomato topped with a quarter cup of tuna fish, drizzled with 2 teaspoons of extra-virgin olive oil, finished with fresh lemon juice and pepper

   MIND foods: Fish, olive oil

   Nutrition: 150 calories, 10 g total fat, 1 g saturated fat, 11 g protein, 5 g carbohydrates, 1 g fiber

6. 3 cups air-popped popcorn, drizzled with extra-virgin olive oil and rosemary

   MIND foods: Whole grains, olive oil

   Nutrition: 170 calories, 10 g total fat, 1 g saturated fat, 3 g protein, 19 g carbohydrates, 3 g fiber

7. Half-cup of cucumber slices combined with a tablespoon of champagne vinegar and pepper

   MIND foods: Vegetables

   Nutrition: 10 calories, 0 g total fat, 0 g saturated fat, 0 g protein, 1 g carbohydrates, 0 g fiber

8. A cup of baby arugula with five sliced strawberries and a tablespoon of balsamic vinaigrette

   MIND foods: Leafy greens, berries, olive oil

   Nutrition: 70 calories, 4 g total fat, 1 g saturated fat, 1 g protein, 7 g carbohydrates, 2 g fiber

9. Half-cup of blueberries mixed with a quarter cup of granola, drizzled with a teaspoon of extra-virgin olive oil

   MIND foods: Berries, whole grains, olive oil

   Nutrition: 190 calories, 6 g total fat, 1 g saturated fat, 3 g protein, 33 g carbohydrates, 3 g fiber

10. Crudités, including 3-inch sticks of carrots (4), red bell pepper (8), and celery (4), with a tablespoon of Dijon mustard

    MIND foods: Vegetables

    Nutrition: 50 calories, 1 g total fat, 0 g saturated fat, 2 g protein, 9 g carbohydrates, 3 g fiber

What's in Season

Foods at peak season are at an ideal stage of quality, taste, and price. This holds true from produce to seafood. For the United States, look at the Best MIND Foods by Season abbreviated guide (page 250) to see what kinds of MIND foods are at their best in each season. It's not comprehensive: the best way to understand what's in season in your specific region is to visit a local farmer's market (https://www.ams.usda.gov/local-food-directories/farmersmarkets).

Frozen and canned (make sure it's in a BPA-free container) are good options to enjoy foods that have been preserved at peak season.

BEST MIND FOODS BY SEASON	
SEASON	**FOODS**
Winter	• Root vegetables and hardy cooking greens like collards and kale • Mushrooms, onions and leeks, potatoes, sweet potatoes and yams, turnips, winter squash • Northern Hemisphere olive oils
Spring	• Strawberries and more delicate greens, from lettuce to string beans and asparagus • Broccoli, cabbage, green beans, lettuce, mushrooms, onions and leeks, peas, spinach • Northern Hemisphere olive oils
Summer	• Berries in general and delicate salad greens • Blackberries, blueberries, cherries, raspberries, strawberries • Wild salmon • Beets, bell peppers, corn, cucumbers, eggplant, garlic, green beans, lima beans, mushrooms, peas, radishes, summer squash, and zucchini • Southern Hemisphere olive oils
Fall	• Hardy vegetables like broccoli and Brussels sprouts • Beets, broccoli, Brussels sprouts, carrots, cauliflower, garlic, ginger, mushrooms, parsnips, pumpkins, sweet potatoes and yams, winter squash • Cranberries • Southern Hemisphere olive oils
Year round	• Dried whole grains • Nuts • Dried beans • Wine • Olive oil • Poultry

MIND Diet At-a-Glance

This is a simple and handy reference sheet for you to come back to or keep with you to remember what to eat (and avoid) on the MIND diet.

WHAT TO EAT	
Every day	• 3 servings of whole grains • 1 serving of vegetables • 1 glass of wine (5 ounces)
Most days	• Leafy green vegetables (6 times per week) • Nuts (5 times per week)
Every other day	• Beans (3 times per week)
Twice a week	• Poultry • Berries
Once a week	• Fish

WHAT TO AVOID	
Less than 1 tablespoon per day	• Butter • Stick margarine
Less than five times a week	• Pastries • Sweets
Less than four times a week	• Red meat
Less than one serving a week	• Whole-fat cheese • Fried fast food

A Dash of Common Sense

Nourishing the body with good nutrition is about the big picture. It is never about single foods or single nutrients. It's about what they add up to and how they work together. This is why nutrition experts promote healthy eating patterns with a balance and variety of many healthy foods. The whole is more important than any parts on their own. While this makes healthy eating a more complex endeavor, it is fundamental to good nutrition. There are a few "rules of thumb" that are fundamental to nutrition that are important to evaluating any diet advice.

There's More Than One Road to Health. There is sound science behind the MIND diet, but even the researchers note that it's the early days for diet-dementia research. For those most concerned about brain health, the MIND diet may do more good than not, and because the diet is based on the Mediterranean and DASH diets, there are many good reasons to follow this eating pattern for heart health and general well-being. Remember, though, that there are other healthy eating patterns, including culturally diverse eating patterns that promote heart health and longevity from East Asia, India, and more.

Sometimes More Isn't Better. A well-established rule in nutrition is that nutrients (and of course the foods that supply them) affect human health in a way that is not linear, which means that more of a good thing isn't always better. Sometimes it's just more, and other times, it's toxic. Instead, it's helpful to think of the way nutrients affect the body's functions as a bell curve. The body can function optimally within a fairly wide range of intake levels, but very low levels lead to deficiencies and very high intakes lead to toxicity. Taking in nutrients at the low or high extremes can interrupt the body's ability to stay healthy, and can even lead to death.

Upgrades Are Essential. Another general rule is that healthy foods must replace unhealthy foods. To add nutritious foods to the diet and keep eating the harmful ones is a step in the right direction, but isn't enough. Similarly, eating healthy foods prepared in unhealthy ways (e.g., frying) doesn't confer the same benefits and can even negate them.

The Best Weight-Loss Diet. Any healthy diet, if followed with the concepts of balance, variety, and portions in mind, should also be ideal for weight management, even when they are not specifically designed for it. The best diet is the one that works for you.

Appendix

Glossary

Alzheimer's disease—Alzheimer's disease is a disease that causes large numbers of nerve cells in the brain to die, commonly marked by memory loss plus cognitive decline in one or more other areas such as language skills, reasoning, attention, or visual perception.

Apolipoprotein E genotyping—Apolipoprotein E (APOE) genotyping is a secondary lab test that may help diagnose late-onset Alzheimer's disease in adults who show symptoms. If a person with dementia also has APOE-e4, it may be more likely that dementia is due to Alzheimer's disease, but it cannot prove it. In fact, there are no definitive diagnostic tests for Alzheimer's disease during life. This test is not appropriate for screening people without symptoms, and some people with APOE e4 will never develop Alzheimer's disease.

Beta-amyloid—The accumulation of beta-amyloid proteins form plaques that eventually disrupt nerve cell function, leading to the death of the affected brain cells, which is believed to be a culprit in Alzheimer's disease.

Cognition—Cognition is the ability to think, learn, and remember. It is the basis for how we reason, judge, concentrate, plan, and organize.

Cognitive decline—Cognitive decline describes the loss of cognitive abilities that occurs as a normal part of the aging process.

It is differentiated from mild cognitive impairment, Alzheimer's disease, and dementia, which are all abnormal conditions.

Dementia—Dementia is not a specific disease. Instead it is the name for a group of symptoms caused by disorders that affect the brain, including Alzheimer's disease and stroke. The most common symptom is memory loss. It is not a normal part of aging.

Dietary Approaches to Stop Hypertension (DASH)—Dietary Approaches to Stop Hypertension (DASH) is a healthy eating pattern developed for research on how diet can reduce blood pressure. It emphasizes eating plenty of vegetables, fruits, and whole grains. It also includes fat-free or low-fat dairy, plus fish, poultry, beans, nuts, and vegetable oils. It discourages foods that are high in saturated fat, such as fatty meats, full-fat dairy products, and tropical oils such as coconut, palm kernel, and palm oils. It also limits added sugar.

Episodic memory—Episodic memory is our personal memory of events at a certain time and place. These memories are specific to each of us and can have an emotional aspect.

Five cognitive domains—The five cognitive domains are: episodic memory, working memory, semantic memory, visuospatial ability, and perceptual speed.

Mediterranean Diet—The Mediterranean Diet is a healthy eating pattern based on traditional foods and beverages from the countries bordering the Mediterranean Sea. Despite variations in the specifics of the foods due to cultural and social differences, key components are fruits, vegetables, whole grains, olive oil, beans, nuts, legumes, seeds, herbs, spices, fish and seafood, with some, but less, poultry, eggs, cheese, yogurt, and occasional wine.

Memory and Aging Project (MAP)—Memory and Aging Project (MAP) is a research study conducted by Rush University Medical Center in Chicago, Illinois, supported by the National Institute on Aging. The study seeks to better understand, treat, and, hopefully, prevent the problems with memory, mobility, and strength associated with abnormal aging.

Mild cognitive impairment (MCI)—Mild cognitive impairment is also referred to as MCI. It is a medical condition that causes people to have more memory problems than other people their age. The signs of MCI are not as severe as those of Alzheimer's disease.

Neuron—Neurons commonly refer to brain cells, though they technically include any nerve impulse–conducting cell in the nervous system, including nerve, brain, or spinal column cells.

Nurses' Health Study—The Nurses' Health Studies (NHS) are among the largest and longest running investigations of factors that influence women's health. Started in 1976 and expanded in 1989, the information provided by the 238,000 dedicated nurse-participants has led to many new insights on health and disease. While the prevention of cancer is still a primary focus, the study has also produced landmark data on cardiovascular disease, diabetes, and many other conditions. Most importantly, these studies have shown that diet, physical activity, and other lifestyle factors can powerfully promote better health. NHS is affiliated with Harvard Medical School, Harvard School of Public Health, Brigham and Women's Hospital, Dana Farber Cancer Institute, Children's Hospital of Boston, Beth Israel Deaconess Medical Center, and Channing Laboratory.

Perceptual speed—Perceptual speed is assessed by the speed of responding (usually using paper-and-pencil tests) with simple content in which everyone would be perfect if there were no time limits.

Semantic memory—Semantic memory refers to a kind of long-term memory that includes knowledge of facts, events, ideas, and concepts.

Visuospatial memory—Visuospatial memory is the ability to understand the spatial relationship between objects. It helps the brain see something and/or its working parts, then understand and replicate it.

Working memory—Working memory is more commonly known as short-term memory, and describes the ability to hold and use information in the moment. For example, doing mental arithmetic.

Recipe Contributors

Individuals

Madeline Basler, MS, RDN, CDN

Ms. Basler is a registered dietitian nutritionist and owner of Real You Nutrition, an integrative nutrition therapy and consulting practice in Long Island, New York. She is a food and nutrition expert, mom, wife, sister, and friend. Her philosophy is to stay authentic and true to ourselves while keeping our body, mind, and spirit healthy so that we can enjoy life to the fullest. She completed her degree in dietetics from Queens College while minoring in journalism, and her master's in nutrition was completed at Stony Brook University in the Department of Family Medicine. She loves to cook for family and friends, eat, chat, and connect with others through healthy food.

Instagram: www.instagram.com/maddybaz
Twitter: www.twitter.com/rdnmaddy
Facebook: www.facebook.com/realyounutrition
Pinterest: www.pinterest.com/realyounutritio
Website: www.realyounutrition.com

Jenna Braddock, MSH, RDN, CSSD, LD/N

Ms. Braddock is a University of North Florida instructor, media spokesperson, blogger, nutrition counselor, recipe developer, and speaker. She regularly appears as a nutrition expert for both TV and print media and believes it is a powerful and fun way to reach people with the message of delicious nutrition. In 2014, Ms. Braddock started the website Make Healthy Easy at www. JennaBraddock.com, where she shares real-life strategies for better health and doable delicious recipes. She also recently joined the team of professionals at the Human Performance Institute as a nutrition coach, where she is excited to help people connect with their life mission and purpose. Ms. Braddock is married to a high school football coach and has two little boys. She loves spending time with her family and will always be found at a football game on Fridays in the fall.

Instagram: www.instagram.com/JBraddockrd
Twitter: www.twitter.com/JBraddockrd
Facebook: www.facebook.com/Jenna-Braddock-
RDN-271368509604284
Pinterest: www.pinterest.com/JBraddockrd
Website: www.JennaBraddock.com

Tracee Yablon Brenner, RD, CHHC

Ms. Brenner is registered dietitian nutritionist and trained culinary professional from Johnson and Wales University. She is the managing partner and culinary director at Triad to Wellness Consulting. At Triad to Wellness, Ms. Brenner works with food companies and commodity boards providing recipe and product development, food quality and product testing, product nutrient analysis, as well as marketing communications and promotional strategy. Ms. Brenner has more than 20 years of experience as a registered dietitian nutritionist and author, working in culinary nutrition, nutrition coaching, and nutrition communications.

Instagram: www.instagram.com/Tracee_RDN_CHHC
Twitter: www.twitter.com/TraceeRDN
Facebook: www.facebook.com/RealFoodMoms
Pinterest: www.pinterest.com/TraceeRDN
Website: www.triadtowellness.com

Amy Gorin, MS, RDN

Amy Gorin is a registered dietitian nutritionist and owner of
Amy Gorin Nutrition. Frequently interviewed by the media, she
privately counsels clients in Jersey City, New Jersey, and New
York City, as well as long distance via virtual counseling. She
works as a motivational speaker and nutrition consultant to
corporations and food companies. Amy has written hundreds of
magazine and Web articles, and authors a nutrition-focused blog
for WeightWatchers.com called *The Eat List*. Her work has been
featured in *Health*, *Women's Health*, *Prevention*, *Dr. Oz the Good
Life*, *Consumer Reports ShopSmart*, Self.com, ReadersDigest.com,
EverydayHealth.com, FitnessMagazine.com, Sonima.com, *Parents*,
American Baby, *Runner's World*, *Yoga Journal*, and more. Amy loves
to spend time in the kitchen, and her recipes have appeared in
Runner's World Meals on the Run (Rodale Books, 2015) and *The
Runner's World Cookbook* (Rodale Books, 2013).
Instagram: www.instagram.com/amydgorin
Twitter: www.twitter.com/amygorin
Facebook: www.facebook.com/amygorin
Pinterest: www.pinterest.com/amydgorin
Blog: www.weightwatchers.com/theeatlist
Website: www.amydgorin.com

Amanda Hernandez, MA, RD

Ms. Hernandez is a registered dietitian, recipe developer, and
blogger at www.nutritionistreviews.com. She lives in Metro Detroit,
Michigan, with her husband Troy, daughter Adalyn, and two
dachshunds. *The Nutritionist Reviews* is a blog that follows her love

for creating healthy recipes, trying new products, nutrition, fitness, and parenting.

Instagram: www.instagram.com/minutritionist
Twitter: www.twitter.com/minutritionist
Facebook: www.facebook.com/minutritionist
Pinterest: www.pinterest.com/minutritionist
Website: www.nutritionistreviews.com

McKenzie Hall Jones, RDN

Ms. Jones is a registered dietitian nutritionist and communications consultant based in Los Angeles. Alongside Lisa Samuel, McKenzie co-owns Nourish RDs, a nutrition communications and consulting company working to deliver clear, actionable nutrition information to clients and the public. She works with agricultural boards and food companies, providing an array of nutrition marketing and public relations services, including social media strategy and management, spokesperson and media outreach, recipe development, and consumer-friendly, evidence-based articles. Additionally, Ms. Jones is a freelance writer and her numerous articles can be found in publications such as *Environmental Nutrition*, the *Chicago Tribune*, *Today's Dietitian*, and more. McKenzie graduated magna cum laude from California Polytechnic State University in San Luis Obispo with a degree in food science and nutrition, and completed her dietetic internship at Bastyr University in Seattle.

Instagram: www.instagram.com/nourishrds
Twitter: www.twitter.com/mckenziehallrd
Facebook: www.facebook.com/nourishrds
Pinterest: www.pinterest.com/nourishRDs
Website: www.nourishRDs.com

Amber Ketchum, MDS, RD

Ms. Ketchum is a registered dietitian nutritionist from San Antonio, Texas. She has bachelor's and master's degrees in nutrition, and has a passion for teaching group nutrition and cooking classes. She started out working in a community setting teaching nutrition to people of all ages, then spent two years working for a weight-loss resort, where she worked with people from all over the world, helping provide nutrition education and strategies to reach their health goals. She is the owner of Homemade Nutrition, LLC, where she does private weight loss consulting, recipe development and nutrition writing for her blog, and teaches group nutrition classes throughout the community. She makes regular appearances on cooking segments for a local morning TV show, where she shares healthy recipes and useful nutrition tips with viewers.

Instagram: www.instagram.com/homemadenutrition

Twitter: www.twitter.com/AmberKetchumRD

Facebook: www.facebook.com/AmberKetchumRD

Pinterest: www.pinterest.com/HomeMadeNutr/

Website: www.homemadenutrition.com

Sarah Koszyk, MA, RDN

Ms. Koszyk is an award-winning registered dietitian and founder of *Family. Food. Fiesta.*, a family recipe and health blog that includes kids' cooking videos. Specializing in weight management and sports nutrition, her lifestyle nutrition program guides people to successfully reach their performance and weight goals in a sustainable, realistic way while still enjoying delicious food for the entire family. Ms. Koszyk also avidly writes and develops recipes. She has authored multiple books, including *Brain Foods: 10 Simple Foods that Will Increase Your Focus, Improve Your Memory, and Decrease Depression*; and *25 Anti-Aging Smoothies for Revitalizing, Glowing Skin.*

Instagram: www.instagram.com/SarahKoszyk

Twitter: www.twitter.com/SarahKoszykRD

Facebook: www.facebook.com/FamilyFoodFiesta

Pinterest: www.pinterest.com/sarahkoszykrd

Website: www.sarahkoszyk.com

Lyssie Lakatos and Tammy Lakatos Shames, RD, CDN, CFT, aka The Nutrition Twins(R)

Ms. Lakatos and Ms. Lakatos Shames are co-owners of NutritionTwins.com and nationally recognized registered dietitians and personal trainers with more than 15 years of experience helping thousands to lose weight, and get healthier, happier, and into tip-top shape. The duo are the authors of *The Nutrition Twins' Veggie Cure*, *Fire Up Your Metabolism*, and *The Secret to Skinny*. They have been featured as experts on major TV networks and popular press ranging from *The Doctors*, *Good Morning America*, *Health*, CNN, and *Fox and Friends* to *USA Today*, *Health Magazine*, and *Vogue*. They have been named as a "Top Influencer" on Pinterest with nearly 4 million followers and they were named in the "Top 20 Nutrition Experts to Follow on Twitter" by *The Huffington Post*. They are experts and bloggers for celebrity Brooke Burke's ModernMom.com as well as for the American Council on Exercise (Acefitness.org) and LIVESTRONG.com. Tammy and Lyssie live in New York City where they enjoy running and biking to keep fit as well as chasing after Tammy's twin daughters.

Instagram: www.instagram.com/nutritiontwins
Twitter: www.twitter.com/NutritionTwins
Facebook: www.facebook.com/The-Nutrition-
    Twins-106607788193
Pinterest: www.pinterest.com/nutritiontwin
Website: www.NutritionTwins.com

Abby Langer, RD

Ms. Langer has been a registered dietitian for 17 years. She runs a successful nutrition media and communications practice in Toronto, Canada. Ms. Langer has been interviewed by many major media outlets in the US and Canada, and her recipes have been published in magazines as well as on her own blog. In her free time, she enjoys running, cooking, and spending time with her husband and two young daughters.

Instagram: www.instagram.com/langernutrition

Twitter: www.twitter.com/langernutrition

Facebook: www.facebook.com/abbylangernutrition

Pinterest: www.pinterest.com/abbyl0724

Website: www.abbylangernutrition.com

Jessica Fishman Levinson, MS, RDN, CDN

Ms. Levinson is a registered dietitian nutritionist and the founder of Nutritioulicious, a New York–based nutrition communications and consulting business with a focus on culinary nutrition. She has extensive experience as a recipe developer, writer, editor, and speaker, maintains the popular *Nutritioulicious* blog, and is the Culinary Corner columnist for *Today's Dietitian Magazine*. Jessica is an active member of the Academy of Nutrition and Dietetics (AND) and various dietetic practice groups of the AND, including Nutrition Entrepreneurs, Food and Culinary Professionals, and Dietitians in Business and Communications.

Instagram: www.instagram.com/jlevinsonrd

Twitter: www.twitter.com/jlevinsonrd

Facebook: www.facebook.com/Nutritioulicious

Pinterest: www.pinterest.com/jlevinsonrd

Website: http://www.nutritioulicious.com

Layne Lieberman, MS, RDN, CDN

Ms. Lieberman is an award-winning culinary nutritionist and author of *Beyond the Mediterranean Diet: European Secrets of the Super-Healthy*. She blogs for *Huffington Post* and WorldRD.com and consults in the food, supermarket, restaurant, and health industries. Ms. Lieberman holds a bachelor of science degree in nutritional biochemistry from Cornell University and a master of science degree in clinical nutrition from New York University. She completed both an internship and fellowship at the Albert

Einstein College of Medicine, and trained at the Culinary Institute of America. She and her husband, Michael, live between New York, Boulder, Colorado, and Vancouver, Canada.

Instagram: www.instagram.com/layneworldrd

Twitter: www.twitter.com/layneworldrd

Facebook: www.facebook.com/WorldRDcom-107899542669682

Pinterest: www.pinterest.com/worldrd

Website: www.worldrd.com

Kara Lydon, RD, LDN, RYT

Ms. Lydon is a nationally recognized nutrition and culinary communications expert and yoga teacher based in Boston. She believes that the secret to a holistically happy life is nourishing the mind, body, and spirit, and she instills this integrative philosophy in the kitchen, yoga studio, working one-on-one with clients, on her food and healthy living blog, *The Foodie Dietitian*, and in her e-book, *Nourish Your Namaste: How Nutrition and Yoga Can Support Digestion, Immunity, Energy and Relaxation* (May 2016). Her blog features delicious seasonal vegetarian recipes and simple strategies to bring more yoga and mindfulness into your life and has been most recently featured on *SHAPE, TODAY, Fitness, SELF, The Kitchn, Prevention*, and Buzzfeed.

Instagram: www.instagram.com/karalydonRD

Twitter: www.twitter.com/karalydonRD

Facebook: www.facebook.com/karalydonRD

Pinterest: www.pinterest.com/karalydon

Website: www.karalydon.com

Jennifer Lynn-Pullman MA, RDN, LDN

Ms. Lynn-Pullman is a Philadelphia-area registered dietitian with a master's degree in nutrition education from Immaculata University. She has worked as a dietitian in many healthcare settings since 2001. Her passion is weight loss and she has spent the last eight years working with several weight-loss surgery programs in the

Philadelphia area. She runs a small private practice in her area and is the owner and author of *Nourished Simply*, a recipe and nutrition blog dedicated to taking the confusion out of eating healthy.
Instagram: www.instagram.com/nourishedsimply
Twitter: www.twitter.com/nourishedsimply
Facebook: www.facebook.com/nourishedsimply
Pinterest: www.pinterest.com/nourishedsimply
Website: www.nourishedsimply.com

Kim Melton, RDN

Ms. Melton is a registered dietitian and owner of NutritionPro Consulting, a Web-based nutrition and counseling business. She also owns and operates a health and wellness blog. She's a mom, a runner, and a nutrition and science writer. She has a passion for educating people on how proper nutrition and a healthy lifestyle can decrease disease risk and improve their lives.
Instagram: www.instagram.com/nutritionpro_1
Twitter: www.twitter.com/NutritionPro_1
Facebook: www.facebook.com/NutritionProConsulting
Pinterest: www.pinterest.com/kimnutritionpro
Website: www.nutritionproconsulting.com

Erin Palinski-Wade, RD, CDE

Ms. Palinski-Wade is "America's Belly Fat Fighter," a nationally recognized nutrition, diabetes, and fitness expert and best-selling author who is known for translating science into understandable sound bites to provide practical information you can use every day. She has contributed her expertise to national media outlets such as *The Dr. Oz Show*, *The Doctors*, *The Early Show*, ABC News, CBS News, Fox News, Food Network, and MSNBC. She operates a private practice in New Jersey and frequently serves as a spokesperson, motivational speaker, and nutrition consultant. She is the author of *2-Day Diabetes Diet*, *Belly Fat Diet for Dummies*, *Walking the Weight Off for Dummies*, *Flat Belly Cookbook for*

Dummies, and is the featured expert on the number-one best-selling diabetes iPad app, Diabetes: What Now?

Instagram: www.instagram.com/erinpalinskiwade

Twitter: www.twitter.com/DietExpertNJ

Facebook: www.www.facebook.com/erinpalinski

Pinterest: www.www.pinterest.com/dietexpertnj

Periscope: DietExpertNJ

Vine: www.vine.co/Erin.Palinski-Wade

Website: www.erinpalinski.com

Sharon Palmer, RDN

Ms. Palmer has created an award-winning career based on combining her two great loves: food and writing. As a registered dietitian with 16 years of healthcare experience, she channels her experience into writing features covering health, wellness, nutrition, cooking, wine, cuisine, and entertainment. She is also a passionate writer about food and environmental issues, having published a number of features on plant-based diets, hunger, agriculture, local and organic foods, eco-friendly culinary practices, sustainability, food safety, humane animal practices, and food security. In particular, Sharon has expertise in plant-based nutrition and blogs every day for her *Plant-Powered Blog*, which received "Top 50 Health Blog" and "Top 100 Nutrition Blog" awards for 2015. Ms. Palmer regularly appears in the media as a nutrition expert, and presents on food and nutrition at venues, including California Dietetic Association, Whole Foods, and Supermarket Symposium all across the country. She also serves as a nutrition advisor to Oldways Vegetarian Network and nutrition editor for *Today's Dietitian*. She serves as a judge for the prestigious James Beard Journalism Award and Books for a Better Life Award.

Instagram: www.instagram.com/sharonpalmerrd

Twitter: www.twitter.com/SharonPalmerRD

Facebook: www.facebook.com/SharonPalmerThePlant
 PoweredDietitian
Pinterest: www.pinterest.com/sharonpalmerrd
Website: www.sharonpalmer.com

Meri Raffetto, RDN

Meri Raffetto is the founder of Real Living Nutrition and author of the *Glycemic Index Diet for Dummies* and coauthor of the *Glycemic Index Cookbook for Dummies, Mediterranean Diet Cookbook for Dummies,* and several "For Dummies" handbooks. She is a recipe developer and has created nutrition programs and education materials for hospitals, private businesses, and employee wellness.
Instagram: www.instagram.com/reallivingnutrition
Twitter: www.twitter.com/realliving2
Facebook: www.facebook.com/RealLivingNutrition
Pinterest: www.pinterest.com/reallivingns
Website: www.reallivingnutrition.com

Vicki Shanta Retelny, RDN, LDN

Ms. Retelny is a nationally recognized lifestyle nutrition expert, and culinary and media consultant. She is the author of *The Essential Guide to Healthy Healing Foods* and *Total Body Diet for Dummies,* which are empowering evidence-based explorations into the landscape of food, encouraging readers to evolve their eating for improved health, happiness, and longevity. As a mother of two, her passion for translating nutrition science into usable, real-life messages combined with her culinary capabilities educates consumers on appreciating healthful ingredients and delicious flavors while creating tasty, nutritious meals. With a particular interest in mindful eating, Vicki's byline has appeared in dozens of national publications. She has appeared on national news programs and regularly contributes to WGN-TV's *Medical Watch.* Vicki lives to eat well in Chicago with her husband, two active youngsters, and their precocious pet pug.

Instagram: www.instagram.com/vsrnutrition
Twitter: www.twitter.com/vsrnutrition
Facebook: www.facebook.com/victoriashanta.retelny
Periscope: vsrnutrition
Website: www.simplecravingsrealfood.com

Chef Allison Schaff, MS, RD, LD

Ms. Schaaf is a food, nutrition, and culinary expert and founder of Prep Dish, a subscription-based gluten-free and paleo meal plan service. She holds a bachelor's degree in culinary nutrition from Johnson and Wales University, a master's in nutrition communications from Tufts University, and became a registered dietitian at New England Medical Center. When she isn't cooking, Ms. Schaaf fully embraces life as an Austinite. She is an avid yogi and enjoys hiking, stand-up paddleboarding, and regular walks around Lady Bird Lake. She enjoys travel and draws culinary inspiration from each trip. Recent adventures include Africa, Australia, and Spain, and frequent trips to Colorado, California, and her home state of Kansas.

Instagram: www.instagram.com/prepdish
Twitter: www.twitter.com/prepdish
Facebook: www.facebook.com/prepdish
Pinterest: www.pinterest.com/prepdish
YouTube: www.youtube.com/channel/UC65ke4V4m2FAMeC6L_
    viVOQ
Website: www.prepdish.com

Amari Thomsen, MS, RD, LDN

Ms. Thomsen is a registered dietitian, recognized nutrition expert, and founder of Eat Chic Chicago. She has experience in nutrition communications and has contributed her expertise to writing articles and developing recipes for a variety of consumer and health publications. She operates a private practice in Chicago and frequently serves as a nutrition spokesperson and public speaker for both media and corporate audiences. Amari specializes in the areas of real food nutrition, recipe development, nutrition education, private and corporate consulting, and content marketing. Amari resides in Chicago, Illinois.

Instagram: www.instagram.com/amarithomsen

Twitter: www.twitter.com/EatChicChicago

Facebook: www.facebook.com/EatChicChicago

Pinterest: www.pinterest.com/EatChicChicago

Website: www.eatchicchicago.com

Christy Wilson, RD

Christy Wilson is a registered dietitian nutritionist and a culinary and nutrition expert based in Tucson, Arizona. She is the founder of Christy Wilson Nutrition consulting service and blog. Ms. Wilson has been in the business of health and wellness as a nutrition counselor, food and nutrition writer, speaker, and cooking teacher since 1999. Christy has written for the Academy of Nutrition and Dietetics, the American Heart Association, and is a contributing editor for *Food and Nutrition Magazine*. *Latina Magazine* named Christy among their Top 10 Latina Health and Fitness Bloggers in 2013, and her expert nutrition advice has been featured in Food Network's *Healthy Eats* blog, *Hey Vivala, The Daily Basics,* and *Latina Magazine*.

Instagram: www.instagram.com/christywil74

Twitter: www.twitter.com/christyschomp

Facebook: www.facebook.com/christywilsonnutrition

Pinterest: www.pinterest.com/christywilsonrd

YouTube: www.youtube.com/channel/
    UCaW42IcPKD2BkTeyp0cEgfA

Website: www.christywilsonnutrition.com

Margot Witteveen, MS, RDN, LD

Ms. Witteveen is a self-described "food nerd" who loves the science of nutrition. This naturally led to her career in dietetics. She holds a master's degree in nutrition from Georgia State University (GSU) and completed her dietetic internship at Southern Regional Medical Center. Her research at GSU was published in *Marathon and Beyond*. Immediately following graduation, she began working at a retirement community and worked with older adults for eight years. During her time there, she became acutely aware of cognitive decline in older adults and how nutrition can have a positive impact on cognition. She then created her private practice Silver Spoons Nutrition in Atlanta, Georgia, a nutrition boutique for women in all capacities. Ms. Witteveen is happiest in the kitchen with her two young boys cooking up delicious recipes for Silver Spoons Nutrition and her family. Margot practices and coaches mindful eating and is perpetually "learning."

Instagram: www.instagram.com/margot_silverspoons
Twitter: www.twitter.com/margotSSN
Facebook: www.facebook.com/silverspoonsnutrition
Pinterest: www.pinterest.com/m_witteveen
Website: www.silverspoonsnutrition.co

Healthy Food Organizations

National Processed Raspberry Council

Created in 2013, the National Processed Raspberry Council (NPRC) represents the processed raspberry industry and is supported by assessments from both domestic producers and importers. NPRC's mission is to conduct nutrition research and promote the health benefits of processed raspberries.

www.redrazz.org

Oldways Whole Grains Council

Oldways is a nonprofit nutrition education organization dedicated to promoting health through cultural heritage and culinary traditions. The Oldways Whole Grains Council is a program of Oldways that helps consumers find whole grain foods and understand their health benefits.

www.oldwayspt.org and www.wholegrainscouncil.org

The Bean Institute

The Bean Institute is owned and managed by the Northarvest Bean Growers Association, an entity created in 1976 as a cooperative effort between dry bean growers in North Dakota and Minnesota. The Bean Institute provides nutrition, health, and culinary information and resources to consumers and home cooks, nutrition and health educators, culinary and foodservice professionals, and school nutrition professionals.

www.beaninstitute.com

U.S. Highbush Blueberry Council

The U.S. Highbush Blueberry Council is an agriculture promotion group, representing blueberry growers and packers in North and South America who market their blueberries in the United States, and works to promote the growth and well-being of the entire blueberry industry. The blueberry industry is committed to providing blueberries that are grown, harvested, packed, and shipped in clean, safe environments.

www.littlebluedynamos.com

Conversions

VOLUME CONVERSIONS	
U.S.	**Metric**
1 tablespoon / ½ fluid ounce	15 milliliters
¼ cup / 2 fluid ounces	60 milliliters
⅓ cup / 3 fluid ounces	90 milliliters
½ cup / 4 fluid ounces	120 milliliters
1 cup / 8 fluid ounces	240 milliliters
WEIGHT CONVERSIONS	
U.S.	**Metric**
1 ounce	30 grams
⅓ pound	150 grams
1 pound	450 grams
TEMPERATURE CONVERSIONS	
Fahrenheit (°F)	**Celsius (°C)**
140°F	60°C
150°F	65°C
160°F	70°C
350°F	175°C
375°F	190°C
400°F	200°C
425°F	220°C
450°F	230°C

Resources

Alzheimer's Disease

Alzheimer's Disease Education and Referral Center (National Institute on Aging): www.nia.nih.gov/alzheimers

Alzheimer's Association: www.alz.org

Family Caregiver Alliance: www.caregiver.org

National Alliance for Caregiving: www.caregiving.org

Food Safety

Be Food Safe: www.befoodsafe.gov

Federal Food Safety Gateway: www.foodsafety.gov

Fight BAC!®: www.fightbac.org

Is It Done Yet?: www.isitdoneyet.gov

USDA Meat and Poultry Hotline: 1-888-MPHotline (1-888-674-6854) TTY: 1-800-256-7072. Hours: 10:00 a.m. to 4:00 p.m. Eastern time, Monday through Friday, in English and Spanish, or email: mphotline.fsis@usda.gov

Visit "Ask Karen," the Food Safety and Inspection Service's Web-based automated response system: www.fsis.usda.gov

Healthy Aging

Administration on Aging: www.aoa.gov

Healthy Aging Program: www.cdc.gov/aging

National Association of Area Agencies on Aging: www.n4a.org

National Institute on Aging: www.nia.nih.gov

Healthy Foods

Academy of Nutrition and Dietetics: http://www.foodandnutrition
.org

The Bean Institute: www.beaninstitute.com

California Olive Oil Council: www.cooc.com

California Strawberries: www.californiastrawberries.com

Cranberry Institute: www.cranberryinstitute.org

Fruits and Veggies More Matters: www.fruitsandveggiesmore
matters.org

International Tree Nut Council Nutrition Research and Education
Foundation: www.nuthealth.org

Monterey Bay Aquarium Seafood Watch: www.seafoodwatch.org

Oldways Whole Grains Council: www.wholegrainscouncil.org

Red Raspberries: www.redrazz.org

U.S. Highbush Blueberry Council: www.littlebluedynamos.com

USDA MyPlate: www.choosemyplate.gov

Wonderful Pomegranate Research: www.wonderfulpomegranate
research.com

References

The references are organized by topic so that you can easily find the right resources to learn more about each one. Since some studies examine more than one food, you may notice that some references appear in more than one section.

B Vitamins

Johnson, L. E. "Vitamin B12." *Merk Manual.* Accessed January 30, 2016. www.merckmanuals.com/home/disorders-of-nutrition/vitamins/vitamin-b-12.

Morris, M. C. "Nutritional determinants of cognitive aging and dementia." *Proceedings of the Nutrition Society,* (2012): 1–13.

Beans

Darmadi-Blackberry, I., M. L. Wahlqvist, A. Kouris-Blazos, et al. "Legumes: the most important dietary predictor of survival in older people of different ethnicities." *Asia Pacific Journal of Clinical Nutrition,* (2004): 217-220.

Shakersain, B., G. Santoni, S. C. Larsson, et al. "Prudent diet may attenuate the adverse effects of Western diet on cognitive decline." *Alzheimer's & Dementia,* (2016): 100-109.

Tsai, H. J. "Dietary patterns and cognitive decline in Taiwanese aged 65 years and older." *International Journal of Geriatric Psychiatry,* (2015): 523-530.

Berries

Bookheimer, S. Y., B. A. Renner, A. Ekstrom, et al. "Pomegranate juice augments memory and fMRI activity in middle-aged and older adults with mild memory complaints." *Evidence-Based CAM*, (2013): 946298. doi: 10.1155/2013/946298

Chen, X., Y. Huang, and H. G. Cheng. "Lower intake of vegetables and legumes associated with cognitive decline among illiterate elderly Chinese: A 3-year cohort study." *The Journal of Nutrition, Health & Aging*, (2012): 549–552.

Devore, E. E., J. H. Kang, M. M. Breteler, et al. "Dietary intakes of berries and flavonoids in relation to cognitive decline." *Annals of Neurology*, (2012): 135-143.

Kang, J. H., A. Ascherio, and F. Grodstein. "Fruit and vegetable consumption and cognitive decline in aging women." *Annals of Neurology*, (2005): 713–720.

Morris, M. C., D. A. Evans, C. C. Tangney, et al. "Associations of vegetable and fruit consumption with age-related cognitive change." *Neurology*, (2006): 1370–1376.

Nooyens, A. C., H. B. Bueno-de-Mesquita, M. P. van Boxtel, et al. "Fruit and vegetable intake and cognitive decline in middle-aged men and women: The Doetinchem cohort study." *British Journal of Nutrition*, (2011): 752–761.

Seeram, N. P., M. Aviram, Y. Zhang, et al. "Comparison of antioxidant potency of commonly consumed polyphenol-rich beverages in the United States." *Journal of Agricultural and Food Chemistry*, (2008): 1415-1422.

Fatty Acids

Martinez-Lapiscine, E. H., P. Clavero, E. Toledo, et al. "Mediterranean diet improves cognition: the PREDIMED-HAVARRA randomised trial." *Journal of Neurology, Neurosurgery, and Psychiatry*, (2013): 1318-1325.

Morris, M. C. "Nutritional determinants of cognitive aging and dementia." *Proceedings of the Nutrition Society*, (2012): 1–13.

Morris, M. C., D. A. Evans, C. C. Tangney, et al. "Fish consumption and cognitive decline with age in a large community study." *Archives of Neurology*, (2005): 1849-1853.

Morris, M. C., C. C. Tangney. "Dietary fat composition and dementia risk." *Neurobiology of Aging*, (2014): S59-S64.

Fish
Larrieu, S., L. Letenneur, C. Helmer, et al. "Nutritional factors and risk of incident dementia in the PAQUID longitudinal cohort." *The Journal of Nutrition, Health & Aging*, (2004): 150–4.

Morris, M. C. "Nutritional determinants of cognitive aging and dementia." *Proceedings of the Nutrition Society*, (2012): 1–13.

Morris, M. C., J. Brockman, J. A. Schneider, et al. "Association of seafood consumption, brain mercury level, and APOE e4 status with brain neuropathy in older adults." *JAMA*, (2016): 315. doi:10.1001/jama.2015.19451.

Morris, M. C., D. A. Evans, C. C. Tangney, et al. "Fish consumption and cognitive decline with age in a large community study." *Archives of Neurology*, (2005): 1849-1853.

Schaefer, E. J., V. Bongard, A. S. Beiser, et al. "Plasma phosphatidylcholine docosahexaenoic acid content and risk of dementia and Alzheimer disease: The Framingham Heart Study." *Archives of Neurology*, (2006): 1545–1550.

Flavonoids & Carotenoids
Harnly, J. M., R. F. Doherty, G. R. Beecher, et al. "Flavonoid content of U.S. fruits, vegetables, and nuts." *Journal of Agricultural and Food Chemistry*, (2016): 9966-9977.

Morris, M. C., C. C. Tangney, Y. Wang, et al. "MIND diet slows cognitive decline with aging." *Alzheimer's & Dementia*, (2015): 1015-1022.

"Vitamin A." *National Institutes of Health*. Last modified February 11, 2016. www.ods.od.nih.gov/factsheets/VitaminA-HealthProfessional.

Lifestyle Guidelines

"About Alzheimer's disease: risk factors and prevention." *National Institute on Aging.* Accessed January 30, 2016. www.nia.nih.gov/alzheimers/topics/risk-factors-prevention.

Barnard, N. D., A. I. Bush, A. Ceccarelli, et al. "Dietary and lifestyle guidelines for the prevention of Alzheimer's disease." *Neurobiology of Aging,* (2014): S74-S78.

"Color additive status list." *FDA.* Last modified December 14, 2015. www.fda.gov/forindustry/coloradditives/coloradditiveinventories/ucm106626.htm.

MIND Diet

Morris, M. C., C. C. Tangney, Y. Wang, et al. "MIND diet associated with reduced incidence of Alzheimer's disease."*Alzheimer's & Dementia,* (2015): 1007-1014.

Morris, M. C., C. C. Tangney, Y. Wang, et al. "MIND diet slows cognitive decline with aging." *Alzheimer's & Dementia,* (2015): 1015-1022.

Nuts

Bao, Y., J. Han, F. B. Hu, et al. "Association of nut consumption with total and cause-specific mortality." *New England Journal of Medicine,* (2013): 2001-2011.

Bes-Rastrollo, M., J. Sabate, E. Gomez-Gracia, et al. "Nut consumption and weight gain in a Mediterranean cohort: the SUN study." *Obesity (Silver Spring),* (2007): 107-116.

Bes-Rastrollo, M., N. M. Wedick, M. A. Martinez-Gonzalez, et al. "Prospective study of nut consumption, long-term weight change, and obesity risk in women." *The American Journal of Clinical Nutrition,* (2009): 1913-1919.

Carey, A. N., S. M. Poulose, and B. Shukitt-Hale. "The beneficial effects of tree nuts on the aging brain." *Nutrition and Aging,* (2012): 55-67.

Martinez-Lapiscina, E. H., P. Clavero, E. Toledo, et al. "Mediterranean diet improves cognition: the PREDIMED-NAVARRA randomised trial." *Journal of Neurology, Nuerosurgery, & Psychiatry,* (2013): 1318-1325.

Mozaffarian, D., T. Hao, H. B. Rimm, et al. "Changes in diet and lifestyle and long-term weight gain in women and men." *New England Journal of Medicine,* (2011): 2392-2404.

Salas-Salvado, J., J. Fernandez-Ballart, E. Ros, et al. "Effect of a Mediterranean diet supplemented with nuts on metabolic syndrome status: one-year results of the PREDIMED randomized trial." *Archives of Internal Medicine,* (2008): 2449-2458.

Valls-Pedret, C., R. M. Lamuela-Raventos, A. Medina-Remon, et al. "Polyphenol-rich foods in the Mediterranean diet are associated with better cognitive function in elderly subjects at high cardiovascular risk." *Journal of Alzheimer's Disease,* (2012): 773-782.

Valls-Pedret, C., A. Sala-Vila, M. Serra-Mir, et al. "Mediterranean diet and age-related cognitive decline: a randomized clinical trial." *JAMA Internal Medicine,* (2015): 1094-1103.

Wengreen, H., R. G. Munger, A. Cutler, et al. "Prospective study of Dietary Approaches to Stop Hypertension—and Mediterranean-style dietary patterns and age-related cognitive change: the Cache county study on memory, health, and aging." *The American Journal of Clinical Nutrition,* (2013): 1263-1271.

Olive Oil

Abuznait, A. H., H. Qosa, B. A. Busnena, et al. "Olive oil derived oleocanthal enhances B-amyloid clearance as a potential neuroprotective mechanism against Alzheimer's disease: in vitro and in vivo studies." *ACS Chemical Neuroscience,* (2013): 973-982.

Estruch, R., E. Ros, J. Salas-Salvado, et al. "Primary prevention of cardiovascular disease with a Mediterranean diet." *New England Journal of Medicine,* (2013): 1279-1290.

Morris, M. C. "Nutritional determinants of cognitive aging and dementia." *Proceedings of the Nutrition Society,* (2012): 1–13.

Valls-Pedret, C., R. M. Lamuela-Raventos, A. Medina-Remon, et al. "Polyphenol-rich foods in the Mediterranean diet are associated with better cognitive function in elderly subjects at high cardiovascular risk." *Journal of Alzheimer's Disease,* (2012): 773-82.

Valls-Pedret, C., A. Sala-Vila, M. Serra-Mir, et al. "Mediterranean diet and age-related cognitive decline: a randomized clinical trial." *JAMA Internal Medicine,* (2015): 1094-1103.

Poultry

"Eat more chicken, fish and beans." *American Heart Association.* Last modified December 2, 2014. www.heart.org/HEARTORG/ HealthyLiving/HealthyEating/Nutrition/Eat-More-Chicken-Fish- and-Beans_UCM_320278_Article.jsp#.VxxI4KODGko

Rurrel, R., and I. Egli. "Iron bioavailability and dietary reference values." *The American Journal of Clinical Nutrition,* (2010): 1461S-67S.

Vegetables and Leafy Greens

Chen, X., Y. Huang, H. G. Cheng. "Lower intake of vegetables and legumes associated with cognitive decline among illiterate elderly Chinese: A 3-year cohort study." *The Journal of Nutrition, Health, & Aging,* (2012): 549–552.

Kang, J. H., A. Ascherio, F. Grodstein. "Fruit and vegetable consumption and cognitive decline in aging women." *Annals of Neurology,* (2005): 713–720.

Morris, M. C., D. A. Evans, C. C. Tangney, et al. "Associations of vegetable and fruit consumption with age-related cognitive change." *Neurology,* (2006): 1370–1376.

Morris, M. C., C. C. Tangney, D. A. Evans, et al. "Fruit and vegetable consumption and change in cognitive function in a large biracial population." *American Journal of Epidemiology,* (2004): S63.

Nooyens, A. C., H. B. Bueno-de-Mesquita, M. P. van Boxtel, et al. "Fruit and vegetable intake and cognitive decline in middle-aged men and women: The Doetinchem cohort study." *British Journal of Nutrition,* (2011): 752–761.

Vitamin E

Morris, M. C. "Nutritional determinants of cognitive aging and dementia." *Proceedings of the Nutrition Society*, (2012): 1–13.

Morris, M. C., J. A. Schneider, H. Li, et al. "Brain tocopherols related to Alzheimer's disease neuropathy in humans." *Alzheimer's & Dementia*, (2015): 32-39.

"Vitamin E." *U.S. National Library of Medicine*. Last modified February 2, 2015. www.nlm.nih.gov/medlineplus/ency/article/002406.htm.

Whole Grains

Hardy, K., J. Brand-Miller, K. D. Brown, et al. "The importance of dietary carbohydrate in human evolution." *The Quarterly Review of Biology*, (2015): 251-268.

Morris, M. C., C. C. Tangney, Y. Wang, et al. "MIND diet slows cognitive decline with aging." *Alzheimer's & Dementia*, (2015): 1015-1022.

Ozawa, M., M. Shipley, M. Kivimaki, et al. "Dietary pattern, inflammation and cognitive decline: The Whitehall II prospective cohort study." *Clinical Nutrition*, (2016). doi: 10.1016/j.clnu.2016.01.013.

Ptomey, L. T., F. L. Steger, M. M. Schubert, et al. "Breakfast intake and composition is associated with superior academic achievement in elementary school children." *Journal of the American College of Nutrition*, (2015): 1-8.

Wine

Estruch, R., E. Ros, J. Salas-Salvado, et al. "Primary prevention of cardiovascular disease with a Mediterranean diet." *New England Journal of Medicine*, (2013): 1279-1290.

Lara, H. H., J. Alanis-Garza, F. E. Puente, et al. "Nutritional approaches to modulate oxidative stress that induce Alzheimer's disease. Nutritional approaches to prevent Alzheimer's disease." *Gaceta Médica de México*, (2015): 229-235.

Noguer, M. A., A. B. Cerezo, E. D. Navarro, et al. "Intake of alcohol-free red wine modulates antioxidant enzyme activities in a human intervention study." *Pharmacological Research*, (2012): 609-614.

Panza, F., V. Frisardi, D. Seripa, et al. "Alcohol consumption in mild cognitive impairment and dementia: harmful or neuroprotective?" *International Journal of Geriatric Psychiatry*, (2012): 1218-38.

Valls-Pedret, C., R. M. Lamuela-Raventos, A. Medina-Remon, et al. "Polyphenol-rich foods in the Mediterranean diet are associated with better cognitive function in elderly subjects at high cardiovascular risk." *Journal of Alzheimer's Disease*, (2012): 773-782.

Index

Recipe Index

Acknowledgments

This book is dedicated to my father, Dr. In E. Moon, the most brilliant person I know. Now in his mid-70s, he is as curious about life as ever, continues to study the latest developments in health and nutrition, maintains his private practice in Newport Beach, spends weekends rock climbing in Joshua Tree, hikes and camps in the mountains, and has been known to run half-marathons at the top of his age class. I credit my curiosity and penchant to go deep on a diverse set of interests to his example.

If my father has shown me how to burn bright, my mother, a chemist by training, taught me how to be steadfast: learning every day, completing what I started, and doing it at the highest level of quality I can muster. Together, they instilled in me the importance of healthy food, being active, and always learning.

This book would not have been possible without my husband, Fred, who set up my standing desk, shared his home office with me, and kept me well supplied with MINDful snacks and hot tea. For support from afar, thanks go to my three sisters and brother, Ahrie, Gurie, Suerie, and Kahmyong, on whom I know I can depend no matter how far we are scattered around this earth.

I'd like to thank the MIND diet research team for devoting previous and ongoing years to the important topic of diet and brain health, the dietitians and healthy food organizations who contributed recipes, and the team at Ulysses Press, especially my editor Casie Vogel and publicist Kourtney Joy for finding me and connecting me to this project.

Last but not least, I'd like to acknowledge all the amazing elders in my life, especially Mom, Dad, Estelle, and Peter, whose wisdom and love of vegetables is inspiring.

About the Author

Maggie Moon, MS, RDN, is a registered dietitian nutritionist and author of *The Elimination Diet Workbook* (Ulysses Press, 2014) and numerous articles for popular health magazines. She has developed curricula for Brooklyn College, New York City after-school programs and providers of continuing professional education for dietitians. Ms. Moon has been profiled in the Academy of Nutrition and Dietetics' book, *Launching Your Dietetics Career* (Eat Right Press, 2011, 2016). She completed her clinical training at New York Presbyterian Hospital of Columbia and Cornell, and holds a master of science degree in Nutrition and Education from Columbia University's Teachers College and a bachelor of arts degree in English from UC Berkeley. She lives in Los Angeles with her husband and a giant shelf of cookbooks.